The Author

A qualified exercise teacher, Rosemary Conley has worked in the field of diet and fitness for over twenty years, but it was in 1986 that she discovered by accident that low-fat eating led to a leaner body.

Forced on to a low-fat diet as a result of a gallstone problem, not only did Rosemary avoid major surgery but her previously disproportionately large hips and thighs reduced dramatically in size.

After extensive research and trials, her *Hip and Thigh Diet* was published in 1988 by Arrow Books. This book and its sequel, Rosemary Conley's *Complete Hip and Thigh Diet*, dominated the bestseller lists for over five years and have sold in excess of two million copies.

Subsequent titles, *Hip and Thigh Diet Cookbook* and *New Hip and Thigh Diet* Cookbook (written with chef and cookery writer Patricia Bourne), *Inch Loss Plan*, *Metabolism Booster Diet*, *Whole Body Programme*, *Shape Up For Summer*, *Beach Body Plan* and *Flat Stomach Plan* have all been instant bestsellers.

Rosemary Conley's *Flat Stomach Plan* was published by Arrow in November 1994 and released on video by V.C.I. in January 1995. Both the book and video shot straight to number one in the respective bestseller charts. Previous fitness videos by Rosemary Conley have total sales exceeding one million copies.

Rosemary has travelled the world promoting her books and appears regularly on television and radio. Since 1990 she has presented her own diet and fitness slot on network television and currently appears on ITV's popular *This Morning* programme.

In 1993 the Rosemary Conley Diet and Fitness Clubs were launched across the United Kingdom. Operating under a franchise system, carefully selected instructors are fully trained to teach the Rosemary Conley philosophy. It is the fastest growing franchise operation in the United Kingdom, with classes proving extremely popular, fulfilling a need to give additional support to followers of Rosemary's diets. It is the first national diet and fitness organisation where only qualified instructors are in operation. In 1995 it won the Franchisor of the Year Award in the 'Newcomer to Franchising' category.

Rosemary lives in Leicestershire with her husband, Mike Rimmington, with whom she runs Rosemary Conley Enterprises and Rosemary Conley Diet and Fitness Clubs Limited. She has a daughter by her first marriage and they are all committed Christians.

BE SLIM!
BE FIT!

WITH

Rosemary Conley

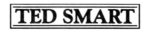

A TED SMART publication 1996

First published in 1995

First published in the United Kingdom in 1995
by Arrow Books Limited
Random House, 20 Vauxhall Bridge Road,
London SW1V 2SA

Random House, Australia (Pty) Limited
20 Alfred Street, Milsons Point, Sydney,
New South Wales 2061, Australia

Random House New Zealand Limited
18 Poland Road, Glenfield,
Auckland 10, New Zealand

Random House, South Africa (Pty) Limited
PO Box 337, Bergvlei, South Africa

Random House UK Limited Reg. No. 954009

ISBN 0091830125

Edited by Jan Bowmer
Designed by Roger Walker
Exercise photography by Martin Spaven
Food photography by Gerrit Buntrock and Andrew Sydenham

Printed and bound in Great Britain by
Butler & Tanner Ltd, Frome and London

Contents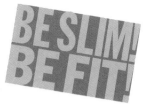

Acknowledgements

This book is based on my column in Yes! Magazine, and I would like to thank everyone involved for their hard work and enthusiasm during my year with the People.

Special thanks must go to Geri Hosier, Assistant Editor (Features) at the People, for her help and encouragement; to her secretary, Vilma Smith, for transforming my scribble into legible print; and to Martin Spaven for his skilful exercise photography.

Very grateful thanks also to Mary Morris, Training and Development Manager at Rosemary Conley Diet and Fitness Clubs, who helped devise the special exercise workouts in this book, which are a modified and expanded version of the ones included in the magazine.

Finally, thanks to Jan Bowmer, who has edited all my books and who has singlehandedly brought together the information from my weekly column in Yes! Magazine to present it in a useful and exciting format for the purposes of this book; to Roger Walker, who designed the inside pages; and to Dennis Barker, Group Design Director at Random House, for the cover design.

Important If you have a medical condition or are pregnant, the diet and exercises described in this book should not be followed without first consulting your doctor. All guidelines and warnings should be read carefully, and the author and publisher cannot accept responsibility for injuries or damage arising out of a failure to comply with the same.

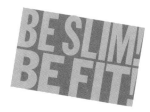

Would you like to be slimmer, healthier, fitter and have more energy and vitality?

Introduction

Yes? Then I'm here to help you with my Be Slim! Be Fit! campaign. In this book I will show you the way to healthy, low-fat eating and sensible exercise through hearty, high-nutrition meals and menu suggestions, plus an easy-to-follow and fun exercise plan.

If you are overweight, you didn't get that way overnight, and achieving a slimmer, healthier body can't be done instantly either. But there is no time like the present to make some positive changes that will transform your figure and your attitude to health and fitness.

Most diets fail because they provide a short-term remedy but not a long-term solution. If you are to lose weight and keep it off, you *must* change the habits that made you overweight in the first place. You'll need to re-educate your shopping trolley, your frying pan and your palate and increase your level of activity, but the more we adopt healthy eating and exercise habits into our everyday lives, the more automatic they become.

Changing the habits of a lifetime will take some willpower, but if you *want* to be slim you'll do it.

We all work better if we have a goal, so decide on a date, or better still, plan your slimming campaign with a deadline in mind – a special occasion such as a wedding, a holiday or celebration that will inspire you into action, and take it one day at a time.

Let's get some objectives clear in our minds. With any weight-loss campaign, we must be realistic. We can't change our height, nor can we alter our basic shape – but we CAN make incredible improvements. We should aim to be lean, not unnaturally thin, and fit, not fanatical. If we reduce the fat in our diet we will reduce the fat on our bodies. Regular exercise will not only help us build muscle, but it will also help us to burn away our fat stores.

The great thing about healthy eating and regular exercise is the almost immediate improvement to our energy levels. This in turn increases our self-confidence and gives us a greater sense of wellbeing, which encourages us to continue so that success is inevitable. But the secret is to keep up those good habits for life.

By following the guidelines and tips in this book you will learn which foods to eat and which to avoid, and how to exercise effectively. On pages 33 to 99 you will find my Be Slim! Be Fit! Eating Plan, which contains a selection of satisfying, low-fat meal suggestions. All you have to do is eat

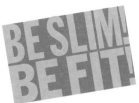

three meals a day, selecting any breakfast, lunch and dinner from the options given.

To help you burn fat, improve your body shape, fitness and energy levels, you can follow my Be Slim! Be Fit! Workout on pages 103 to 129. There's also a special Five-minute Workout for those days when time is at a premium, plus a stretch routine which will help improve your flexibility and range of movement.

Getting fitter is like investing in a deposit account. The more we put in, the greater the rewards. In other words, the more physical activity we do, the more energy we have. It's wonderful. By combining a nutritious, low-fat diet with regular exercise the results can be staggering. Follow the advice and tips, and in just a few weeks you will notice a real difference in the way you look and feel. If you don't need to lose weight but just want to eat healthily, you can still follow the meal suggestions but increase the quantities a little and enjoy the occasional additional indulgence.

By making a low-fat diet and regular exercise part of your everyday lifestyle you will reap enormous benefits. So, make a commitment to achieve a leaner body and a healthier lifestyle – it's never too late to start. Go for it – you have nothing to lose but inches.

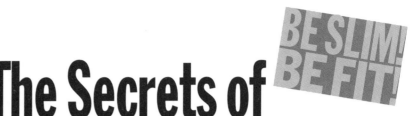

The Secrets of Successful Slimming

Why is it that when we've just tried on that dress we bought last year and can't believe how tight it is, and we promise ourselves 'That's it. I am DEFINITELY going to be good now' that we find ourselves devouring some highly fattening food?

It is because we panic and our bad feelings about ourselves send us reaching for the first thing to comfort us in such traumatic moments – namely FOOD! Instant, sweet, fatty food. Why? Well, I'm afraid our mums were probably to blame.

When we were children and fell down and hurt ourselves or had to take some ghastly-tasting medicine, we were comforted by some sweet food treat – and old habits die hard. It's as simple as that.

So what is the answer?

If someone were to offer you a new wardrobe of clothes or the holiday of a lifetime if you lost all your unwanted weight by a certain date, you wouldn't be questioning whether you *could* do it. You just would. Suddenly the rewards would be worth the sacrifices and you'd be happy to make the necessary changes to your lifestyle for you to succeed.

What you need is a goal – a reason for losing your excess pounds. Just fancying being slimmer is not enough. You need an occasion or a holiday to inspire you, to provide you with a date for which you can aim. If you don't have anything planned, invent something – a treat or an outing. Put a date in the diary and keep it in mind – all the time! Try and devise something that involves your partner and family too. If they will benefit from your success, they'll support you all the way.

Be realistic about your goal. We can't change our basic shape, so the best alternative is to work hard at making the best of what we have and not underestimate the improvements that we can make to our body shape, weight and energy levels. And by setting ourselves continuous goals, each time we achieve one, no matter how small it is, our confidence is increased and we feel able to accomplish even more.

Achieving a slim and healthy body can't be done instantly. The only way to shift the fat forever is to make gradual, long-term progress. But if you stick with it, I promise you WILL see results. Just follow the guidelines in this book, and you'll see how simple it is.

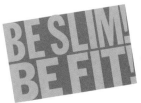

What We Need for a Healthy Diet

It's now proven that a low-fat diet is the healthiest and most effective way to lose weight. You can eat more than on most other diets because fat contains twice as many calories as protein foods such as chicken, meat or fish, or carbohydrates such as bread, potatoes, rice or pasta.

Low-fat eating doesn't have to be painful or boring, or mean that you have to go without your favourite foods. Cooking without fat is easier than you may think. There are now so many low-fat alternatives on the supermarket shelves that it's easy to cut down on the fat and still eat a varied diet without sacrificing the flavour.

Food is like the fuel in our cars. We need food for energy to enable our bodies to function. If we eat too much, we store the excess as fat. If we eat less than our bodies need, this causes the body to draw upon its fat stores to make up the difference.

But food does more than just supply energy. It provides the essential nutrients necessary for good health. Just as a car needs oil, water, grease, brake fluid and polish, we need a variety of foods too to enable us to achieve maximum performance. Each day we need a balanced supply of nutrients (protein, carbohydrates, vitamins, minerals and fat) to enable our bodies to function properly and efficiently – to keep the heart pumping, organs operating, tissue and bones growing and repairing, and a million and one other functions.

We can obtain all the nutrients we need from a varied diet without adding any extra fat or oil since we only need a small amount of fat in our daily diet. Even the leanest cuts of meat, poultry and fish contain fat, and providing we eat a varied diet we are unlikely to be deficient. In particular, the oil found in fish such as mackerel, tuna and salmon is of significant nutritional value, and I recommend that these be eaten once or twice a week. Since vegetarians won't be obtaining fat from meat, fish and poultry, they can add a few nuts and seeds to their diet and even a few drops of oil to their cooking. On the next page I have included some guidelines for vegetarians who wish to follow a weight-reducing diet.

Each day we should eat at least 6 oz (150 g) of protein food. Protein is found in meat, fish, poultry, cottage cheese, beans and pulses. We need lots of vegetables and, as these are low in calories and fat, they can be eaten freely at mealtimes. In addition, we need around 12 oz (300 g) of fruit a day, so I recommend you drink a $1/4$ pint (125 ml) fruit juice at breakfast and add a piece of fruit with other meals.

We get most of our energy from carbohydrates such as cereal, bread, potatoes, rice and pasta, and these foods should form the basis of your

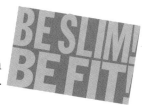

diet. If you are trying to lose weight, keep to the quantities described in the meal suggestions, since eating too many of these – or indeed of anything – despite their low fat content will cause you to gain weight.

Dairy products are a good source of calcium, and by selecting low-fat varieties of yogurts, fromage frais and cottage cheese we can still obtain sufficient calcium while reducing the fat content. Indeed, skimmed and semi-skimmed milk actually contain more calcium than full-cream milk.

Vegetarian Dieting

A vegetarian diet excludes red and white meat, fish, poultry and animal fats but does not exclude dairy products (unlike a vegan diet, which excludes all animal-related produce, including dairy products.) Here are some guidelines on creating a nutritious and balanced, low-fat vegetarian diet.

A healthy vegetarian diet offers an excellent combination of plenty of fresh fruit and vegetables, which boost the fibre content of the diet, plus an overall low fat intake, since most ingredients have a low fat content.

The diet is based on five major food groups, which vegetarians should regularly incorporate into their daily diet. These are:

Grains: barley, buckwheat, millet, oats, rice, rye, wheat.
Pulses: beans, lentils, peas.
Nuts and seeds: any kind of nuts; sesame seeds, poppy seeds, caraway seeds, sunflower seeds. (Generally, nuts and seeds are high in fat but are allowed in moderation in a vegetarian diet to compensate for the lack of fat from meat.)
Dairy products: low-fat cottage cheese, fromage frais or yogurt, skimmed or semi-skimmed milk.
Fruits and vegetables: selection of all kinds.

The first four groups are rich in protein, but they are not complete proteins in themselves and therefore need to be combined in the following ways (see right).

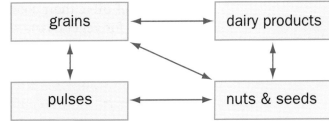

Combining these food groups together in a meal and in the course of the day will ensure you receive an adequate supply of protein.

This might seem daunting at first, but if you mix and match you'll

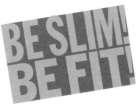

soon see how easy it is. A breakfast of muesli with yogurt or milk (grains and dairy products), a light lunch of sesame Ryvitas, salad and cottage cheese (seeds, grains, vegetables and dairy) and an evening meal of vegetarian spaghetti bolognese made using soya mince and spaghetti (pulses and grains) is an example of how this can be achieved.

Eat More to Weigh Less

When we think of losing weight, we tend to think in terms of eating less, but, in fact, if we are to lose weight successfully and keep it off for good we need to eat sufficient food to help keep our metabolism buoyant.

Our metabolism is the mechanism within our bodies that effects a chemical breakdown of the foods we eat and results in the utilisation of the nutrients the body needs to carry out repairs, renewal and growth as well as to generate the energy we need to cope with everyday activities.

The metabolic rate is the rate at which the body burns up calories. A calorie is a unit of heat, and that heat provides energy. The more energy we expend, the hotter we become and the more calories we burn up. This is where exercise can help to accelerate weight loss.

However, the majority of calories are automatically utilised by the body to renew and repair body tissue, to grow our hair and nails, and to provide enough energy for the heart to pump blood around the body to supply all the oxygen we need non-stop throughout our entire life. The amount of energy (calories) our body needs for these functions alone is determined by our individual basal metabolic rate (bmr).

The average basal metabolic rate of a woman is about 1,400 calories per day, and for a man it is approximately 1,800. The basal metabolic rate can be increased by regular physical activity. Generally speaking, the average bmr of men is subject to greater variance than that of women, proportionate to the degree of physical activity involved in their daily work. The bmr can also be reduced, not by a lack of exercise, but by a reduced calorie intake.

If the body receives insufficient calories the bmr will reduce to a level that will still fulfil the body's basic physiological needs. It is therefore essential for slimmers to keep their bmr as high as possible by eating sufficient calories – around 1,400 to 1,500 calories a day for women, and 1,800 to 1,900 for men.

It is easy to lose weight on this intake of calories because from the moment we get out of bed in the morning we start to use calories in addition to those used by our bmr for basic bodily functions. The extra

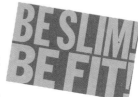

energy we need will be supplied from the excess fat stored in the body. This principle forms the basis of any weight-reducing diet.

It is a complete fallacy to think that the less food you eat, the more weight you lose. Each person's metabolic rate responds to the amount of food they eat. If we eat too little, it slows down and the body's ability to burn fat is greatly reduced. This is Nature's way of protecting us against future starvation. If the body does not receive sufficient food, it goes into 'emergency' mode and compensates by holding on to the small amount of food it does receive and converts it to reserves of fat, instead of using it for energy, in case the food supply is cut off completely.

This is just what the dieter wants to avoid, since it reduces the body's effectiveness at converting fat into energy, preferring to store it as fat for a rainy day! And although we might register a weight loss on the scales, we wouldn't be losing fat. What we would be losing is water and lean muscle tissue, which could leave us looking gaunt and flabby. Then as soon as we returned to our normal pattern of eating, we would put all the weight back on plus more, because our metabolic rate will have fallen, and therefore our bodies will require less food than before to function – a disaster for any slimmer. This is why those who follow very-low-calorie or meal-replacement-type diets often end up weighing more than they did in the first place.

The secret of successful slimming therefore is to give your body plenty to eat in the form of high-bulk, low-fat, nutritious foods and not to cut the calories too low. So, eat three meals a day and eat sufficient at mealtimes to satisfy your appetite. Eating regular and normal-sized meals and taking regular exercise will help us lose body fat and keep the metabolic rate buoyant.

Without doubt, one of the main reasons for the incredible success enjoyed by followers of my low-fat diets has been the simplicity – foods that are easy to buy, meals that are easy to prepare and eating plans that are easy to follow.

Perhaps most important of all, my dieters don't go hungry. I try to select foods that are high in nutrition but low in fat and, where possible, foods with maximum volume, thus enabling the greatest possible exercise for the jaws! Food that requires a great deal of chewing not only makes us feel we are eating more, but inevitably we eat it more slowly. This allows time for the food to reach the stomach before we have finished eating and gives us a better chance of knowing when we have eaten enough. In addition, foods that require a lot of chewing also usually take a fair bit of digesting. And if the digestive system has to work harder, it helps us burn more calories.

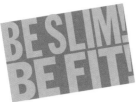

Learn to Handle the Difficult Times

For a slimming campaign to be successful in the long term it is important to make some changes in your day-to-day life. The food that made you overweight in the first place, and the lack of activity that made you lethargic and unfit must be considered as part of your past.

In times of weakness or depression, it is the instant foods that appeal. Depending on whether you have a sweet or savoury tooth, it's the biscuits, cakes, sweets, chocolate and ice cream or the crisps, peanuts and cheese – or for some people all of them – that seem irresistible. Recognise what your weaknesses are and try not to have these foods in the house.

Learn to anticipate the bad times. Many women find that pre-menstrual tension plays havoc with their diet and that the craving for something sweet seems uncontrollable. At such times, make sure the refrigerator is stocked up with diet drinks and diet yogurts or fromage frais to help keep the damage to a minimum.

If you do find yourself 'cheating' don't get so disheartened that you throw in the towel. Just acknowledge that small lapses will not cause a huge amount of damage and, providing you get straight back on track you'll be able to repair the damage very quickly. The next day try to be more physically active to compensate.

Getting into a three-meals-a-day routine will help reduce your chances of 'cheating'. Eating sufficient at mealtimes will mean you are less tempted to nibble between meals. Try having a long diet drink before you start eating and this will help you feel fuller more quickly. We need to learn as many tricks as possible to help us stay on the straight and narrow, but remember – we are only human after all!

Finally, realise that sometimes we need to indulge, but if we restrict our indulgences they will do little harm. They just slow down our weight-loss progress.

What to Do When the Scales Seem to Stick

Wouldn't it be great if we knew that, providing we stuck rigidly to a diet, we would lose, say, two pounds (1 kg) every week? But our bodies are not machines. We are all unique. I have a lady who attends my diet and fitness club and who never strays from the diet, but she usually stays the same weight for three weeks and then loses four or five pounds (1.8–2.3 kg) in the fourth week. She has lost a magnificent six stone (38 kg) and has come to terms with her spasmodic progress.

Other people can go for weeks at the same weight and then, if they

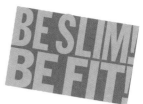

persevere, the weight suddenly starts to shift. Why does the body reach a plateau when, no matter how hard we try, the scales just seem to stick and our metabolism appears to be on a 'go slow'?

There is no simple answer, but here are some tips to get the weight shifting again.

We can jolt our metabolism by increasing (yes, that's right, *increasing*) our food intake slightly so that the body is convinced we're not dieting. Going out for a meal could do the trick.

Another method is to make the body work harder to digest the food we eat by breaking up the daily menu into a greater number of, but smaller, meals. Just as a car burns more fuel when it is used for lots of short journeys, the same principle applies to our bodies. Each time you eat, the whole digestive mechanism sets to work. That uses energy and therefore burns more calories. So try splitting your usual three meals a day into six mini meals.

For instance, here is a sample basic diet menu:

Breakfast: 1 oz (25 g) cereal with milk and sugar plus 1 banana.
Lunch: 4 Ryvitas topped with Marmite and 4 oz (100 g) cottage cheese and salad, plus 5 oz (125 g) diet yogurt.
Dinner: 4 oz (100 g) lean meat plus 16 oz (400 g) vegetables and gravy, followed by 1 meringue basket with strawberries and fromage frais.

You can divide this three-meal menu into six smaller meals by eating the 'second course' two to three hours after the first course. The diet menu would then look like this:

Breakfast: 1 oz (25 g) cereal with milk and sugar.
Mid-morning snack: 1 banana.
Lunch: 4 Ryvitas topped with Marmite and 4 oz (100 g) cottage cheese.
Mid-afternoon snack: 5 oz (125 g) diet yogurt.
Dinner: 4 oz (100 g) lean meat plus 16 oz (400 g) vegetables and gravy.
Evening snack: 1 meringue basket with strawberries and fromage frais.

Be careful not to eat a greater amount of food in total. This tip only works if you are strict about the quantities you eat.

You should also increase your level of physical activity. Choose an activity that is reasonably energetic such as going for a bike ride, a swim or a gentle jog – something that will make you slightly out of breath for 15 to 20 minutes. This will increase the metabolic rate and keep it elevated for several hours. Try this for a week and see if it gets *your* weight moving.

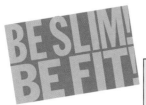

Ten Tips For Successful Weight Loss

Follow these ten simple rules and you will be on the way to a trimmer and healthier body.

1 Eat three low-fat meals a day, selecting from the breakfast, lunch and dinner suggestions in this book.

2 Stop cooking with fat. Using non-stick pans and utensils will help.

3 Always use fat-free or low-fat products instead of full-fat varieties. Stop using butter, margarine or low-fat spreads on bread. Instead, use very low-fat or fat-free dressings and sauces.

4 Use skimmed or semi-skimmed milk in place of full-fat (silver top) milk, except for children up to the age of seven years.

5 Do not eat between meals but eat sufficient at mealtimes to satisfy your appetite. Fill up on extra vegetables with your evening meal if necessary to prevent hunger pangs later.

6 Use artificial sweeteners instead of sugar in drinks, or reduce by 50 per cent the amount of sugar you normally take.

7 Drink low-calorie drinks in place of ones high in sugar. Having a couple of long, soft drinks before your evening meal will help you feel full more quickly.

8 Restrict your alcohol intake to a maximum of two drinks per day for men and one drink for women. Do not save these up and have them all in one go, as too much alcohol taken in one session will convert to fat on your body.

9 Eat enough! If you eat too little your metabolism will slow down. You need to eat 1,400 to 1,500 calories a day to achieve optimum weight loss.

10 Enlist the support of family or friends to encourage you in your campaign for a leaner, fitter body. Or better still, persuade them to join you. There's no doubt that dieting and exercising with others helps keep the willpower flowing. Joining a local club (see page 160) and mixing with others who are just like you – who understand the misery of being overweight and who desperately want to do something about it – has proved to be a successful way of keeping that willpower going.

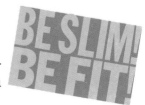

Finally, don't cheat at all. Each time you finish off the children's leftovers or lick the spoon covered with the cake mixture, you're taking a step backwards.

Don't get despondent if your progress is slow. Stick at it, and then one day when you're least expecting it, you'll lose several pounds and you'll realise that all the effort was worthwhile. Remember, you only fail at something if you stop trying.

After we have settled into a new eating routine we don't continue to lose weight at the same rate as at the start of our campaign, but we do continue to lose inches, and when the inches disappear it is a clear indication that the fat is being burned away. So don't be disheartened if your weight loss is not as great as you thought it would be – it is the inches that really count.

We often fall into the trap of not appreciating just how much progress we have made. A good way to remind ourselves is to keep a plastic bag or an old supermarket carrier bag handy. Each week when you weigh yourself, fill the bag with packets or cans of food weighing the equivalent of the weight you have lost.

As the weight piles into the bag, lift it up every now and then and remind yourself of your progress and just how much weight you have actually lost. This is a real memory jogger and a great stimulant to encourage you to continue.

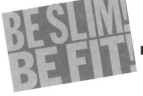

Take Active Steps to Get Fit

The benefits of regular exercise are enormous. Not only does it help us to get fitter and healthier, it also relieves stress, burns fat, improves our body shape and speeds up the whole process of weight and inch loss. However unfit or unused to physical activity we are, we can increase our fitness level relatively quickly if we exercise regularly.

Consider carefully how you can start increasing your level of physical activity and aim to do something physical each day. No matter how little, it all adds up to help us slim down and tone up. Even if it's only ten minutes a day it will make a significant difference to how you look and feel.

The crucial factor is to find a form of exercise you enjoy. If you haven't exercised for years, DON'T go and have a game of squash or try and jog for five miles. Instead go for a brisk walk or go swimming – start gently and gradually increase the frequency, intensity and duration of the activity. Walking is now acknowledged as the best form of all-round exercise. Wear sensible shoes and stride out as often as possible.

Take every opportunity to incorporate activity into your everyday lifestyle. Park your car at the furthest point rather than the nearest. Take the stairs not the lift. Walk the children to school instead of driving them. Increase your activity level in any way you can – it all adds up to a fat-burning, fit-making workout.

Remember, *regular* exercise is the key. It helps us burn fat and tone up so that even when we are resting, our body is more efficient at burning fat. And we don't have to do less physical activity as we get older. In fact, the more physically active we are, the younger we look and feel. It truly is a win-win situation.

Exercise shouldn't be a chore but should form part of our everyday lives, so it has to be enjoyable. Make the effort. It's worth it. And whether we're mowing the lawn, cleaning the windows or clearing out the shed – it's all good exercise. Look upon these tasks as a workout, not as chores, and you won't mind doing them half as much!

In addition to increasing your activity level, pay attention to your posture. To stand in a good posture you should stand tall, pull your tummy in and your shoulders back and down. Aim to do this as often as possible throughout the day so that it becomes a habit. The more upright

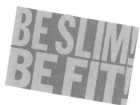

we are, the younger we look. So, whether you are standing in a bus queue or at the sink, practise, practise and practise some more!

For optimum benefits in terms of weight loss and body reshaping we need to do a combination of different kinds of exercise. Aerobic exercise (exercise that makes us breathe faster and more deeply) will help us burn fat. Toning exercises will help us build muscle, and the more muscle we have, the higher our metabolic rate and the more calories we burn. We need to undertake both types of exercise in order to maximise our weight loss and our long-term weight maintenance and fitness levels.

When we lose fat off our bodies, we literally burn it off, just like burning a log on a fire. It disappears into the air and makes heat – and that's what WE do. Exercise combined with low-fat eating helps us to lose FAT *without* losing lean muscle tissue and at the same time ensures that our fat stores are not replenished. Toning exercises will help increase our lean muscle tissue. But don't worry, it would be highly unlikely for a woman to build the kind of muscle we see on body builders, so you won't end up looking like a weight lifter.

Aerobic Exercise

'Aerobic' simply means 'with oxygen', and aerobic exercise is any activity that makes us slightly out of breath and forces more oxygen into the body, making our heart and lungs work harder and become stronger – activities such as brisk walking, gentle jogging, swimming, cycling, step or aerobics classes. It will also improve our general health and fitness as well as encouraging oxygen to the skin, which gives us a healthy glow. Aerobic exercise may conjure up images of 'going for the burn' and working out so hard that we're pouring with sweat and ready to drop. However, this is not the way to achieve maximum fat burning and a level of fitness that can greatly improve the standard of our health and the quality of our lives. Fitness is about being able to cope with the demands placed upon us in everyday life and having sufficient energy in store to cope with emergencies.

In order for aerobic exercise to be effective, it has to be sustained for a minimum of 15 to 20 minutes and carried out at a moderate level (not to the point of exhaustion) so that you are mildly perspiring and a little out of breath. At this level the body calls upon its fat stores for fuel. But don't overdo it. You should still able to carry on a conversation.

Aim to do some form of aerobic activity every day if possible. Choose an activity or activities that you enjoy so that you are more likely to continue to do them. Always warm up first, by starting very gently and

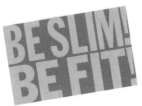

gradually build up the activity. It is important to slow down at the end to cool off before you stop and to bring the heart rate back down to normal.

Toning Exercises

Toning exercises work in a different way and rely on the strength (pulling power) of the muscles and their endurance (staying power). Working a muscle strongly and performing a sufficient number of repetitions to allow it to become slightly fatigued causes that muscle to recruit extra muscle fibres, which increases the shape and the size of the muscle. Muscle requires fuel to sustain it while fat requires virtually none, so if the body has more muscle than fat, it will require more calories to maintain it, which will lead to an increased metabolic rate. This is good news for slimmers as it means we can burn more calories just going about our everyday lives.

On pages 103 to 129 you will find my Be Slim! Be Fit! Workout, a simple but effective exercise routine that combines aerobic and toning exercises to help maximise your fat loss and improve your body shape, fitness and energy level. In addition, there is a Five-minute Workout consisting of a short tone and stretch routine, which is useful on those days when you find your schedule is particularly hectic.

The stretches on pages 125 to 129 will help improve your flexibility and range of movement, so try to practise these as often as possible even on those days when you don't have time to do the full Be Slim! Be Fit! Workout.

You Are Never Too Young to Start

If children or teenagers are athletic by nature and participate regularly in sport, that's terrific. They are unlikely to have an overweight problem as the number of fat cells that we take into adulthood is determined during our early years, and the more physically active we are as teenagers, the fewer fat cells we have.

While this number of fat cells is determined at a comparatively early age, they will of course fill up or empty according to our daily diet and physical activity. With this in mind it is clear to see that educating our families towards a healthy lifestyle will greatly help prevent obesity problems later, so children should not be brought up on a diet of chocolate and chips and video games.

Instead, encourage healthy eating and more physical activity. Children should be encouraged to play games such as hide-and-seek,

TAKE ACTIVE STEPS TO GET FIT

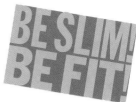

rounders, or skipping. Develop themes for the younger ones, for instance, marching like soldiers, training to be a footballer, or dancing to music – anything, but make it fun! Start being more active as a family. Go on a bike ride or go swimming. Play outdoor games or go for a walk or a picnic.

Age is No Barrier

I am often asked if exercise is still good for us when we get older. Without exception, exercise will help us stay fitter, look younger and enable us to remain independent. And research has proved it's never too late to start.

In one trial the progress of exercise students in their twenties was compared with that of mature students in their eighties. All progressed at exactly the same rate.

Trials have also been undertaken in residential care homes for the elderly. In one trial, after much persuasion, the elderly residents joined in the exercises and performed them from their chairs. Within a very short period of time they responded positively, with increased mobility, enhanced mental awareness and a significant improvement in attitude. They all look forward to their exercise class now.

One of my ladies, Marjorie, has been attending my diet and fitness club for thirteen years. She has lost three stone (19 kg) and works out every week. She is eighty-eight years old but looks more like seventy. Marjorie is able to look after her husband, dig the garden and cut the hedges. She attributes her youthfulness to her regular exercise – and who am I to argue?

So what happens to our bodies as we get older? Basically, they become more fibrous, which means they lose flexibility, and the muscles become weaker. This is a perfectly natural process and we can't stop it – but we can slow it down. Performing the stretches from the cool-down section on pages 125 to 129 will help improve flexibility and give you a greater range of movement, which is particularly useful for older people. If we can do up our own dress zips and bend down to tie our own shoelaces, we stay more independent. The key is to keep moving. Any activity is better than none, so don't use age as an excuse!

Exercising with Equipment

How many of us have sometimes been tempted to invest in a gadget or piece of equipment which we believe will help give us a beautiful sylph-like form? There's the massage glove that promises cellulite-free legs,

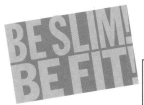

Ten Tips For a More Active Lifestyle

Follow these ten simple rules and you will be on the way to a trimmer and healthier body.

1 Get up 15 minutes early and do ten minutes exercise BEFORE you shower and dress for the day. It's tough the first couple of mornings, but you quickly get into the new habit and you'll feel so good you'll keep it up.

2 Find an activity that you enjoy and that is practical. For instance, you can't go jogging in the dark or work out if your partner is trying to sleep, but you could work out quietly to a fitness video in the living room or walk around the garden or local park or just around the block.

3 Walking (or running) up and down stairs is an easy way to give yourself a good cardiovascular workout. Adopt a good posture, don't rush it and do wear cushioned trainers.

4 Make a list of all the physical jobs you can do in a day. For example, walking the dog, vacuuming the carpet, hanging out the washing, walking to the shops, walking the children to school. See how many more you can add to your list. The more you do, the fitter you will feel.

5 Make it a rule never to use the lift (unless you are carrying something heavy).

6 Always park your car in the furthest space, not the nearest.

7 When you walk anywhere, try to increase the pace and feel the extra effort you are investing. It will pay greater dividends.

8 Learn to play again – anything. Remember the games you played as a child and start playing them with your children or grandchildren. It's fun.

9 Always adopt a good posture. Practising good posture habits will have a dramatic effect on your stature, your figure and will keep you looking younger.

10 Remember, getting physically fit means more than just losing weight and looking better. We fight infection more easily, we have lots more energy and we enjoy life much, much more! So do it!

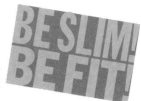

body wraps that promise to dissolve our unwanted pounds, and pills and potions that claim to increase our metabolic rate. If only it were that simple and they really did work. But the truth is they don't.

Don't be fooled by the lissom model illustrating the virtues of these 'miracle' products. You can bet your life she's never even needed them. There are no short cuts, no instant solutions. Just as a face cream won't change our faces, no pills, potions, wraps or rubber massagers will change our body shape.

But we tend to like gadgets and, if chosen carefully, exercise equipment can be helpful – but only if you use it regularly.

Using an exercise bike, rowing machine or stepper can be monotonous, so the answer is to pedal, row or step while watching your favourite TV programme or soap. This way, you won't get bored and the programme times ensure you do a regular workout. If you have more than one piece of equipment, do five minutes on each. This adds variety and works different muscles, which is even better.

Here is a brief overview of some of the most popular home exercise equipment.

Exercise Bike: This gives a good cardiovascular (aerobic) workout and specifically works the calves and thighs. Pedal at a steady pace for maximum fat burning.

Rowing Machine: Again, this gives a good cardiovascular workout and specifically works the legs, arms and shoulders. Row at a moderate pace for maximum fat burning.

Steppers: The little steppers, which cause the feet to rise and fall only a few inches, are not much use, as the range of movement is insufficient to create a useful workout. The more substantial model (with handlebars) is excellent and offers a much greater range of movement for the legs. It gives a good cardiovascular workout, is a good fat burner and can really help tone your seat, hips and thighs.

Mini Trampoline: This gives a good cardiovascular workout, but you need a reasonable sense of balance and should learn a variety of moves to make the workout fun. Work at a level that enables you to achieve mild breathlessness in order to burn fat.

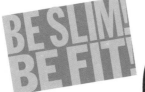

Getting Started

If we want to lose weight and get fitter we need to make a conscious effort to scrap unhealthy bad habits and create healthy good ones. Establishing good habits takes self-discipline. We have to make some real changes in our shopping list, food preparation, eating and exercise habits. When shopping for food we need to check the labels and select low-fat brands. We also have to decide how we are going to become more active whether it's playing sport, jogging, working out at home or going to the gym or a fitness class.

To set yourself off on your Be Slim! Be Fit! campaign, start by re-educating your refrigerator and store cupboard. Read carefully the Traffic Light Guide to low-fat eating. Use up all the high-fat foods you already have in the house and next time you go shopping replace them with low-fat alternatives listed in the Green list. Getting our minds into gear to lose weight is 90 per cent of the battle, and removing those tempting foods from the kitchen will help enormously.

Many potential slimmers are put off by the prospect of having to purchase expensive, exotic foods for themselves while the rest of the family continue with their 'normal' foods. The beauty of low-fat eating is that it can actually be cheaper. You don't need to buy anything extra – you just don't buy certain foods such as butter, oil, cream, mayonnaise, pies and pastries. Instead, stick to healthy, low-fat foods which are readily available, high in nutrition and low in fattening power.

To save extra money, go shopping towards the end of the day in supermarkets where fresh produce is often reduced as the 'best before' date is due to expire. Prices on market stalls are usually cheaper than in the supermarkets because the overheads are considerably less. As closing time approaches, most of the produce is virtually given away to clear the stall before it's time to pack up. There's no doubt that real bargains are to be enjoyed by those who look for them.

If you have to cook on a budget, experiment with beans and pulses. These are nutritious and tasty and help the housekeeping money go further.

Eating low-fat foods is good for the rest of the family too (except for very young children), so there is no need to eat in isolation. Children under the age of seven should never be placed on a weight-reducing diet as they need extra energy to make them grow. Nevertheless, encouraging the children to eat healthily will set them up with good habits for life.

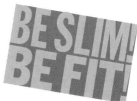

Use your imagination when preparing packed school lunches. Invest in a good lunch box that will incorporate your child's favourite yogurt. Experiment with any leftovers such as pizza or pasta. Cold pizza tastes great and pasta twirls mixed with low-fat salad dressing and tuna is delicious.

Try cutting sandwiches into fun shapes using a biscuit cutter. Follow a theme each day and include some carrot sticks with the rabbit-shaped sandwiches or cut everything into circles or chip shapes. Include chopped apple with raisins and chopped marshmallow in a little container.

Add a pot of yogurt or fromage frais. Peel and chop an orange to make it easier to eat and more appetising. Use your imagination, but think 'healthy'.

READY! STEADY! GO!
Your Traffic Light Guide to Foods

The following foods are high in fat and should be kept to a minimum within the family diet. Some exceptions are made for vegetarians. While an occasional treat is acceptable for those not wishing to lose weight, high-fat foods can be addictive and lead to overweight later.

- All butters, margarines, low-cholesterol or low-fat spreads or any similar products (except those containing 4% fat or less).
- Cream, soured cream, whole milk, Gold Top.
- Lard, oil (all kinds), dripping, suet.
- Fried foods of any kind, except dry-fried.
- All cheese, except low-fat cottage cheese and fromage frais.
- All nuts, except chestnuts (vegetarians may eat small quantities of nuts).
- Sunflower seeds (vegetarians may eat small quantities).
- Goose and all fatty meats.
- Fat or skin from all meats and poultry.
- Meat products, e.g. sausages, salami, pork pie, faggots, black pudding, haggis, pâté.
- Egg products, e.g. Scotch eggs, crêpes, quiche, pancakes, custards, Yorkshire pudding.
- All sauces and dressings containing cream, whole milk or eggs, e.g. salad dressing, mayonnaise, French dressing, parsley sauce, cheese sauce, Hollandaise sauce.

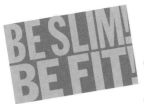

- Cakes, sweet biscuits, pastries (including savoury pastries), sponge puddings etc.
- Chocolate, toffees, fudge, caramel, butterscotch.
- Savoury biscuits and crispbreads (except rye crispbreads).
- Lemon curd.
- Marzipan.
- Cocoa and cocoa products, except very low-fat brands.
- Crisps (including low-fat crisps).
- Cream soups.
- Avocado pears.
- Ice cream made with real cream, e.g. Cornish.

Food in the Amber list is moderately low in fat and offers healthy options for the whole family and the occasional treat for those on a diet.

- Biscuits: water biscuits.
- Cakes: low-fat sponge cakes (e.g. Swiss roll), Jaffa cakes, scones without butter, buns without cream.
- Cheese: low-fat Cheddar, Edam or Gouda.
- Condiments: tartare sauce
- Dressings: reduced-oil salad dressings.
- Drinks: low-fat versions of Horlicks, Ovaltine or drinking chocolate.
- Eggs: except fried.
- Fish: kippers, rollmop herrings, eels, sardines, bloaters, sprats.
- Jams and preserves.
- Meat: low-fat sausages well grilled, grilled lean bacon, grilled beefburgers.
- Milk: whole milk with cream removed.
- Puddings: ice cream (not creamy Cornish varieties), pancakes made with skimmed milk, trifle made with fat-free sponge and custard made with skimmed milk, served without cream.
- Soups: any brand.
- Yogurts: non-diet varieties.
- Yorkshire pudding: made with skimmed milk and cooked in a non-stick pan.

Items on the Green list are low in fat or virtually fat free and therefore ideal for everyone, particularly those people who are trying to lose weight. However, quantities do count, so follow my guidelines within the meal suggestions.

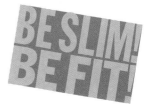

- Beans, lentils, pulses: any type.
- Bread: any type without fat (not fried or buttered).
- Breakfast cereal: any type.
- Cakes: very low fat.
- Cheese: low-fat brands of cottage cheese and fromage frais.
- Condiments: any type except tartare sauce.
- Crispbreads: rye crispbread, Ryvita.
- Dressings: oil-free and fat-free dressings, yogurt dressing, vinegar, lemon juice.
- Eggs: egg whites can be eaten freely, but limit egg yolks to a maximum of two per week.
- Fruit: any type of fresh, frozen or tinned fruit, except coconut and olives; fruit juices and dried fruit in moderation.
- Game: any type, roasted without fat and with all skin removed.
- Gravy: made with gravy powder or low-fat granules.
- Ice cream: Wall's 'Too Good To Be True'.
- Jams and preserves: marmalade, jam, honey and syrup – all in moderation.
- Meat: lean red meat (twice a week maximum) cooked without fat.
- Meat substitutes: textured vegetable protein, vegeburgers.
- Milk: skimmed or semi-skimmed.
- Nuts: chestnuts only.
- Offal: any type in moderation, cooked without fat.
- Pasta: egg-free varieties.
- Pickles and relishes: any type in moderation.
- Poultry: chicken, duck, turkey – all cooked without fat and with all skin removed.
- Prepared meals for slimmers: Boots, Lean Cuisine, Menu Plus, Weight Watchers ranges.
- Puddings: custard made with skimmed or semi-skimmed milk; fresh fruit salad; jelly; meringues; rice pudding made with skimmed or semi-skimmed milk; low-fat varieties of yogurt.
- Rice: brown rice, boiled or steamed.
- Sauces: Barbecue, apple, cranberry, horseradish, brown, mint, soy, Worcestershire, tomato ketchup, mustard, yeast extract, white sauces made with skimmed milk and no fat, low-fat cook-in-sauces.
- Soups: clear and non-cream varieties.
- Soya: low-fat type.
- Stuffing: made with water.
- Sugar: any type in moderation; artificial sweeteners.

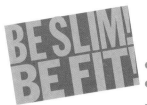

- Vegetables: any type (except avocado) cooked and served without fat.
- Yogurt: low-fat varieties; avoid Greek.

Shopping Tips

- When shopping, always make a list and stick to it. Don't be seduced by clever marketing ploys aimed at tempting you to buy foods you don't need.
- Always check the nutrition panel on food products. If anything contains more than 4 grams of fat per 100 grams of the total weight, leave it on the supermarket shelf. The only exceptions are meat, fish and poultry and foods that you will use sparingly such as curry powder or mustard.
- Beware of misleading labels. A product labelled 'low fat' may still be high in fat. Low-fat spreads are a classic example.
- Stock up on low-fat cook-in-sauces. They are tasty and quick and easy to use.
- Buy canned, chopped tomatoes to add to dishes. They are just as nutritious and much more convenient than trying to chop up plum tomatoes.
- Always select low-fat brands of yogurts, fromage frais and cottage cheese. If in doubt, check the nutrition panel for fat content. Beware of brands with added cream.
- Where possible, choose wholemeal products in preference to refined ones when buying bread, rice, pasta etc.
- When buying canned fish such as tuna always check it is canned in brine not oil.
- Choose the leanest cuts of meat and chicken and avoid those which have been prepared in breadcrumbs.

The Low-down on Low-fat Cooking

Low-fat cooking is so easy once you get into the habit. Once you know which low-fat foods you can exchange for what, you can make up your own recipes and modify your old favourites. Think about what you are cooking. If a recipe calls for fatty ingredients, consider which items you can substitute to reduce the fat content.

Also, think of alternative methods of cooking which don't require fat. Treat yourself to a good non-stick frying pan and learn to dry-fry foods instead of frying in butter or oil. Just preheat the pan and add the meat or vegetables. Any food can be cooked this way.

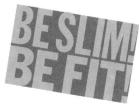

If grilling or roasting meat, always use a wire rack to allow the fat to drain away. Try cooking chicken (with skin removed) in a covered casserole or in aluminium foil 'parcels' to help retain the flavour and moisture.

Remove any visible fat from steak, chops and chicken BEFORE cooking. Use 'cook in' readymade sauces to add flavour and moisture to meat and vegetables and you won't miss the fat.

Top Ten Cooking Tips

1 Cook without fat at all times. Using non-stick utensils enables you to cook perfectly without it.

2 Placing a lid on a saucepan or frying pan during cooking encourages more moisture into the dish being prepared and aids thorough cooking of the food.

3 Remove all skin and fat from chicken and meat BEFORE cooking to avoid the flesh soaking up the fat.

4 Learn to adapt your favourite recipes by substituting low-fat ingredients. For instance, use cornflour mixed with cold water as a thickener instead of a butter and flour roux. Use low-fat yogurt in place of single cream, and low-fat fromage in place of double cream, but be sure never to overheat these products.

5 When cooking vegetables, rice or pasta, add a stock cube to the water to add extra flavour. And don't throw the water away, it can be used as a stock or soup later.

6 The flavour of some recipes will be further enhanced by allowing the dish to stand after cooking and then reheating it thoroughly before serving.

7 Dishes such as kebabs benefit from marinating in a sauce for an hour or two BEFORE cooking. This enables the flavours to penetrate the meat and enhance the taste.

8 When cooking mince, always dry-fry first and then drain the fat from the pan before adding other ingredients. Each ounce of fat you drain away is fat that won't reach your hips!

9 Use lots of low-fat sauces and dressings to spice up your food. HP, barbecue, tomato, mushroom, soy and chilli sauces are all low in fat.

10 Make gravy with Bisto, Marmite or Bovril, plus cornflour to thicken if necessary. Avoid gravy granules unless they are the low-fat variety. Never use meat juices, unless you have first drained off ALL the fat.

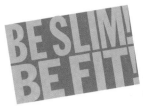

Utensils You Will Need

- Non-stick frying pan with a lid
- Non-stick saucepans with lids
- Spatula and spoons compatible with non-stick utensils
- Measuring jug
- Garlic press
- Chopping board and sharp knife
- Kitchen weighing scales
- Tablespoon and teaspoon for measuring

Store Cupboard

The following items are useful to have in the store cupboard as they are common ingredients or accompaniments in low-fat recipes.

- Arrowroot
- Black pepper in a pepper mill
- Branston pickle
- Brown sauce
- Canned mushrooms
- Canned tomatoes
- Cereals
- Chilli and garlic sauce
- Chilli powder
- Cook-in-sauces (low-fat brands)
- Cornflour
- Curry powder
- Dried low-fat milk
- Garlic powder
- Gravy powder or low-fat granules
- Ground ginger
- Herbs and spices (any kind)
- Horseradish sauce
- Lemon juice
- Mint sauce
- Mixed dried herbs
- Mustard (French and English)
- Pasta (egg-free)
- Raisins
- Reduced-oil salad dressing
- Rice (preferably brown)
- Salt

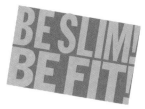

- Stock cubes (beef, chicken, vegetable and fish)
- Sultanas
- Tomato ketchup
- Tomato purée
- Vinegar
- White wine vinegar
- Yeast extract

Regular Items for the Refrigerator

- Diet drinks
- Diet yogurts
- Low-fat fromage frais
- Low-fat natural yogurt
- Orange juice (unsweetened)
- Salad dressings (very low-fat or fat-free brands)
- Semi-skimmed or skimmed milk
- Sparkling mineral water
- Tomato juice

The Be Slim! Be Fit! Plan – How It Works

Decide on a date when you will begin your new Be Slim! Be Fit! campaign. Do take the time and trouble to weigh and measure yourself carefully as you progress, particularly at the start of your campaign and enter the details on the chart on page 158. Scales should be placed on a flat board for greatest accuracy and should not be stored in the bathroom where they are likely to be affected by damp. Keeping a weekly record of your progress enables you to look back and see how well you have done and this will encourage you to continue.

Before you begin, ask your partner or a friend to take a 'before' photograph of you. Once you have achieved your new slimline figure, you'll look back at this photograph with pride. Watch how you turn that unfit and untoned body into a youthful and energetic life-machine.

From now on, increase your activity level and get into the habit of eating three low-fat meals a day – and don't nibble in between meals. If you maintain these lifestyle changes you will never regain the weight you lose.

Follow the instructions in The Be Slim! Be Fit! Eating Plan on pages 33 to 39 and select from the breakfast, lunch and dinner meal suggestions provided. Develop the habit of enthusing about your new eating plan and picture yourself succeeding.

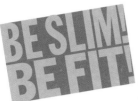

Practise the Be Slim! Be Fit! Workout 0n pages 103 to 129 on as many days of the week as possible. This will help burn fat and tone you up as you lose inches. In addition, try to do some form of aerobic activity each day such as brisk walking, swimming or cycling for a minimum of 15 to 20 minutes. On those days you don't have time to do the full workout, try the Five-minute Workout for an effective mini tone and stretch routine, or practise the stretches on pages 125 to 129 since these form a good flexibility routine. If you plan your fitness schedule in advance and make a note in your diary, you'll do it. If you just wait until you feel like it, you never will. When we've actually done it we feel brilliant – so make a date NOW.

Try to put maximum energy into everything you do throughout each day. Just being more active will enable you to increase your fitness level, but think how much more you could benefit if you performed the Be Slim! Be Fit! Workout on a regular basis AND combined it with an increased activity level in your everyday life. The improvements will be even greater and will happen much more quickly. Re-read pages 18 to 23 for more ideas on increasing your level of activity. Don't forget to involve the rest of the family too.

My Be Slim! Be Fit! eating plan is easy to follow and it won't leave you feeling hungry or deprived. Just follow the instructions below and choose from the meal suggestions provided. Make sure you vary your choices in order to receive a balanced intake of nutrients. The meal suggestions and recipes and suitable for all the family, so there's no need to eat in isolation. There are quick and easy options throughout as well as recipes that take a little more preparation.

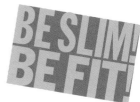

The Be Slim! Be Fit! Eating Plan

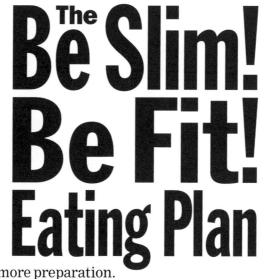

Don't forget to combine this eating plan with a programme of regular exercise and feel the extra energy as the fat melts away.

Diet Instructions

Eat three meals a day, selecting one meal from the Breakfast, Lunch and Dinner suggestions on the following pages. For dinner you are allowed three courses: a starter, main course and dessert. If you prefer, you can save your starter or dessert to have as a snack later in the evening.

Do not eat between meals, but if you feel really peckish, fill up on sticks of carrots, celery, cucumber and peppers.

Men over 5 ft 0 in (1.78 m) or who are involved in heavy physical labour may increase the quantities by 25 per cent.

It is important that you avoid foods on the Red list (see pages 25 to 26) during your weight-loss campaign. Once you have reached your target weight you may be able to indulge in some of these foods occasionally.

Daily Allowance

$^1/_2$ pint (250 ml) skimmed or semi-skimmed milk
One alcoholic drink for women, two for men
$^1/_4$ pint (125 ml) unsweetened orange juice

Drinks

Tea and coffee may be drunk freely providing the skimmed or semi-skimmed milk allowance is not exceeded. Use artificial sweeteners in place of sugar whenever possible.

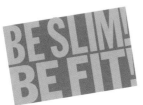

Men may drink two alcoholic drinks per day and women one drink. One drink means a single measure of spirit or one glass of wine, or a small glass of sherry or $^1/_2$ pint (250 ml) beer or lager. If using mixers, always ensure these are 'slimline'. Diet drinks may be drunk freely. For those who do not drink alcohol, an additional fruit juice may be consumed daily.

Drink as much water as possible throughout the day.

Daily Nutritional Requirements

In devising your menus, each day try to incorporate the following *minimum* quantities:

6 oz (150 g) protein food (fish, poultry, meat, cottage cheese, baked beans)
12 oz (300 g) vegetables (including salad)
12 oz (300 g) fresh fruit (including fruit juice)
6 oz (150 g) carbohydrate (bread, cereals, potatoes, rice, pasta)
$^1/_2$ pint (250 ml) skimmed or semi-skimmed milk

I would also suggest you take one multivitamin tablet each day to make doubly sure that you are getting all the vitamins you need, but providing you eat a varied diet you should obtain sufficient nutrients.

Diet Notes

- Unlimited vegetables includes potatoes as well as all other vegetables provided they are cooked and served without fat.
- Pasta and rice may be substituted for potatoes. Use 2 oz (50 g) uncooked weight as a serving guide per portion.
- Limit egg yolks to a maximum of two per week. The whites can be eaten freely.
- Red meat should be restricted to just two helpings per week.
- Gravy may be taken with dinner menus provided it is made with gravy powder or low-fat granules. Do not add meat juices from the roasting tin unless you first discard the fat.
- One piece fresh fruit means one average apple or one orange etc., or approximately 4 oz (100 g) any fruit such as grapes, pineapple, strawberries etc. Do not eat fruit between meals.
- For adults milk should be skimmed or semi-skimmed. 'Silver top' milk is acceptable providing the cream is removed.
- Diet yogurt means low-fat, low-calorie brands. If it is difficult to find low-fat brands of natural yogurt, try to select brands without added cream.

THE BE SLIM! BE FIT! EATING PLAN

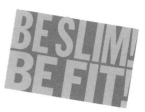

- Cottage cheese and fromage frais should be the low-fat varieties. Flavoured varieties are acceptable, but check the nutritional panel for fat content and avoid ones with added cream.
- Bread should be wholemeal whenever possible. For guidance, one slice of regular bread from a large thin-sliced loaf weighs 1 oz (25 g). A slice from a large medium-sliced loaf weighs 1¹/₂ oz (37.5 g). Unless otherwise specified, one slice equals 1 oz (25 g).

Your Quick and Easy Diet

To start you on the road to successful slimming here is a quick a easy diet which does not require any special recipes.

Breakfasts

- 1¹/₂ oz (37.5 g) any cereal plus ¹/₄ pint (125 ml) milk in addition to allowance.

  OR

- 2 oz (50 g) toast spread with 4 teaspoons marmalade.

  OR

- 2 pieces any fresh fruit plus 2 x 5 oz (2 x 125 g) diet yogurts.

Lunches

- 8 oz (200 g) jacket potato topped with 8 oz (200 g) baked beans or 3 oz (75 g) cottage cheese and salad.

  OR

- 4 slices Slimcea or Nimble spread with ketchup, fat-free dressing or pickle and made into sandwiches with salad and any of the following:
  2 oz (50 g) chicken, turkey or lean ham.
  3 oz (75 g) tuna in brine.
  3 oz (75 g) cottage cheese.

  OR

- ¹/₂ pint (250 ml) home-made soup plus 2 slices wholemeal bread.

  OR

- 5 pieces any fresh fruit.

  OR

- 1 slimmers' cup-a-soup, 2 pieces fresh fruit and 2 x 5 oz (2 x 125 g) diet yogurts.

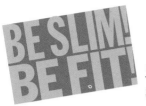

Dinners

Select a starter, main course and dessert.

Starters

- ¹/₂ fresh grapefruit.

  OR

- ¹/₂ pint (250 ml) consommé or any clear soup.

  OR

- Wedge of melon.

Main Courses

Select one of the following and serve with unlimited vegetables and potatoes.

- 8 oz (200 g) white fish.

  OR

- 6 oz (150 g) chicken, turkey or duck with skin removed and weighed without bone.

  OR

- 4 oz (100 g) lean red meat.

  OR

- 4 oz (100 g) lean pork.

Desserts

- 8 oz (200 g) any fresh fruit.

  OR

- 2 x 5 oz (2 x 125 g) diet yogurts.

  OR

- 4 oz (100 g) fresh fruit plus 5 oz (125 g) diet yogurt.

  OR

- 2 brown Ryvitas topped with 3 oz (75 g) cottage cheese.

  OR

- 3 oz (75 g) Wall's 'Too Good To Be True' ice cream.

> The following conversion rates have been used throughout this book:
> 1 oz = 25 g; 1 fl oz = 25 ml; ¹/₂ pint = 250 ml.

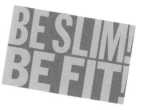

Breakfasts

SELECT ANY ONE

Quick and Easy Breakfasts

- 2 oz (50 g) wholemeal roll spread with horseradish sauce and filled with 2 oz (50 g) smoked turkey breast and 2 fresh tomatoes, sliced.
- 4 brown Ryvitas spread with 4 teaspoons marmalade, plus 5 oz (125 g) diet yogurt.
- 2 oz (50 g) wholemeal roll spread with mustard and filled with 2 oz (50 g) wafer-thin ham.
- 2 oz (50 g) wholemeal roll spread with 2 teaspoons honey, plus 5 oz (125 g) diet yogurt.
- 4 brown Ryvitas spread with pickle and topped with $1^1/_2$ oz (37.5 g) wafer-thin chicken, turkey or ham.
- 4 brown Ryvitas spread with Marmite and topped with 4 oz (100g) cottage cheese.
- 1 slice wholemeal toast spread with 2 teaspoons marmalade, plus 2 pieces fresh fruit.
- 1 slice wholemeal toast spread with 2 teaspoons marmalade, plus $^3/_4$ oz (18 g) cereal with milk from allowance and 1 teaspoon sugar.
- 2 slices wholemeal toast spread with 4 teaspoons marmalade.
- $^1/_2$ oz (12.5 g) branflakes with 1 banana, sliced, plus 5 oz (125 g) diet yogurt.
- 5 oz (125 g) diet yogurt plus 2 bananas.
- 1 wholemeal muffin or 1 bagel spread with 2 teaspoons jam, plus 1 piece fresh fruit.

Ryvitas spread with pickle and topped with wafer-thin ham

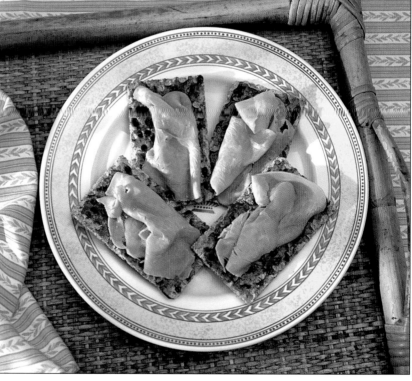

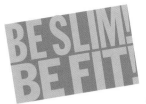

Cereal Breakfasts

- $1\frac{1}{2}$ oz (37.5 g) Fruit and Fibre cereal with $\frac{1}{2}$ teaspoon sugar and milk from allowance.
- 1 oz (25 g) any cereal with 1 teaspoon sugar and milk from allowance, plus 5 oz (125 g) diet yogurt.
- 1 oz (25 g) Rice Krispies and 1 chopped banana with milk from allowance and $\frac{1}{2}$ teaspoon sugar.
- 1 oz (25 g) Special K, plus 4 oz (100 g) strawberries, served with milk from allowance and 1 teaspoon demerara sugar.
- 1 oz (25 g) Special K mixed with 10 sultanas and 5 oz (125 g) natural yogurt, plus 1 teaspoon sugar.
- 1 oz (25 g) All Bran plus 1 chopped pear or banana served with milk from allowance and 1 teaspoon demerara sugar.
- 1 oz (25 g) All Bran mixed with 6 oz (150 g) chopped melon and served with milk from allowance.
- $1\frac{1}{2}$ oz (37.5 g) muesli topped with 4 oz (100 g) fresh fruit mixed with diet yogurt.
- 2 Weetabix with milk from allowance and 2 teaspoons sugar.

Home-made Austrian Muesli

SERVES 1

1 eating apple
$\frac{1}{2}$ oz (12.5 g) oats
$\frac{1}{2}$ oz (12.5 g) sultanas
$\frac{1}{2}$ banana
2 teaspoons bran
Milk from allowance *or*
3 oz (75 g) natural yogurt
Honey (optional)

Grate or chop the apple, chop the banana, then mix all the ingredients together and add honey to taste if required.
Alternatively, mix all the ingredients (except the banana) together the night before and leave to soak overnight in skimmed milk. Add the chopped banana before serving.

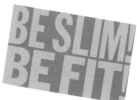

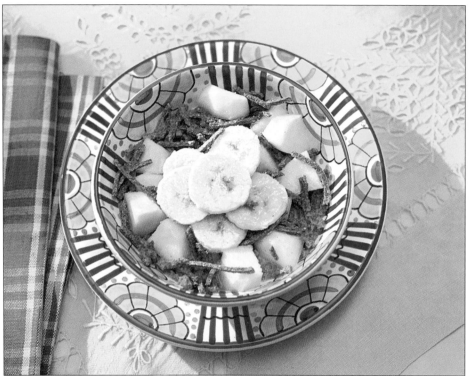

All Bran with chopped
pear and banana

Special K with
strawberries

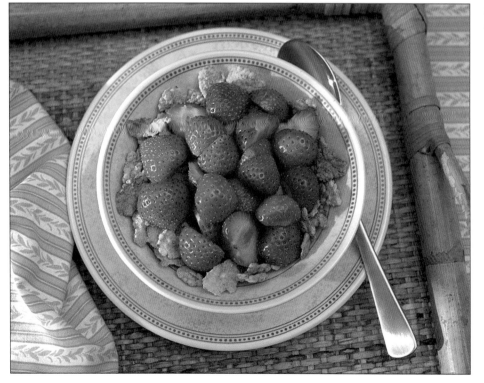

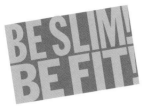

Fruit Breakfasts

- 8 oz (200 g) fresh fruit salad with 2 x 5 oz (2 x 125 g) diet yogurts.
- 5 prunes soaked in black or fruit tea overnight, plus 5 oz (125 g) diet yogurt.
- Melon balls in slimline ginger ale, plus 1 slice toast spread with 1 teaspoon marmalade.

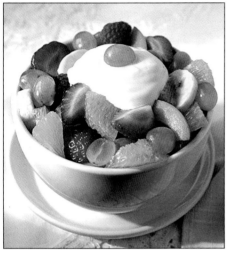

Fresh fruit salad with diet yogurt

- 4 pieces fresh fruit (e.g. a banana, an orange, a pear and 4 oz/100 g strawberries).
- 4 oz (100 g) tinned peaches in natural juice, plus 5 oz (125 g) diet yogurt.
- 10 oz (250 g) fresh fruit salad plus 2½ oz (62.5 g) fromage frais.
- 10 grapes mixed with 6 oz (150 g) chopped melon and 5 oz (125 g) diet yogurt.
- 5 fresh plums plus 5 oz (125 g) diet yogurt.
- 3 green figs (fresh or canned) with 5 oz (125 g) diet yogurt.
- Dried Fruit Compote: Soak 2 prunes, 2 apricots and 10 sultanas in a fruit-flavoured herbal tea overnight. Serve cold.
- Banana Milkshake: Place 1 chopped banana and 2 teaspoons clear honey in a blender. Whisk until smooth. Add 7 fl oz (175 ml) semi-skimmed milk and blend for a further minute.

Pineapple Boat

SERVES 2

1 medium-sized fresh pineapple
8 oz (200 g) seasonal fruit of your choice
10 oz (250 g) diet yogurt
2 strawberries to decorate

Divide the pineapple into two halves from top to bottom. Do not cut away the leaves (they add to the decorative look). Cut away the flesh with a grapefruit knife then cut into cubes, removing the hard core.

Prepare the remainder of the fruit by washing and cutting into bite-sized pieces and mix with the pineapple. Pile the fruit into the hollowed-out pineapple halves and dress with the yogurt.

Decorate each with a strawberry and serve chilled.

Peach Brûlée

SERVES 2

6 oz (150 g) peaches canned in natural
juice, drained
6 oz (150 g) fromage frais
2 tablespoons demerara sugar

Switch the grill on to full heat. Place the
drained peaches in two ovenproof
ramekin dishes.

Cover the peaches with the fromage
frais. Sprinkle one tablespoon sugar
over each dish to cover the top. Place
under the hot grill, watching
continuously, and remove from the grill
as soon as the sugar caramelises.

Cheese and Apricot Pears

SERVES 4

4 ripe pears
Lemon juice
8 oz (200 g) cottage cheese
4 tablespoons apricot jam or preserve

Peel the pears, cut in half lengthways
and remove the core. Brush with lemon
juice to prevent discolouration.

Fill the cavities with the cottage
cheese mixed with the apricot jam or
preserve.

Serve chilled.

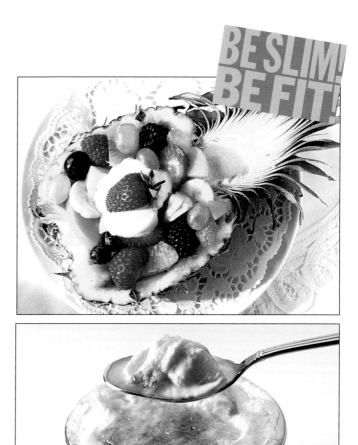

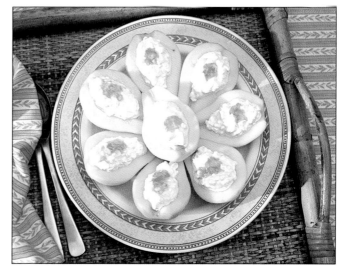

From top to bottom:
Pineapple Boat
Peach Brûleé
Cheese and Apricot Pears

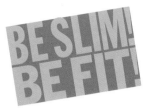

Cooked Breakfasts

- 1 slice wholemeal toast plus 5 oz (125 g) baked beans.
- ½ grapefruit, 1 oz (25 g) grilled lean bacon with unlimited tomatoes and grilled mushrooms.
- 2 slices Nimble or Slimcea topped with 4 oz (100 g) baked beans and 8 oz (200 g) canned tomatoes.
- 1½ oz (37.5 g) (dry weight) porridge made with water and served with milk from allowance and 1 teaspoon honey.
- 1 oz (25 g) lean ham, 2 grilled fresh tomatoes, 4 oz (100 g) baked beans, ½ slice wholemeal toast (no butter).
- 1 poached egg on 1 slice wholemeal toast (no butter), 1 sliced tomato, plus small glass orange juice.
- ½ fresh grapefruit plus 1 boiled egg and 1 slice wholemeal toast (no butter).
- ½ fresh grapefruit plus 1 poached egg on 1 slice wholemeal toast (no butter).
- 1 whole grapefruit, 1 lean rasher bacon, grilled, plus 2 slices Nimble or Slimcea spread with mustard or tomato ketchup.
- 8 oz (200 g) smoked haddock, microwaved or steamed, served with 1 slice Nimble or Slimcea.
- Crispy Bacon and Beans on Toast: Chop 1 lean rasher bacon into small pieces and dry-fry lightly. Add a little chopped onion and continue to cook gently. Add 3 large tablespoons baked beans, mix and warm through. Serve on 1 slice wholemeal toast (no butter).

Crispy Bacon and Beans on Toast

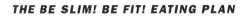

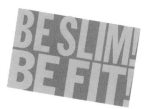

Ham, tomatoes and baked beans with
$^1/_2$ slice toast

Smoked haddock
with 1 slice bread

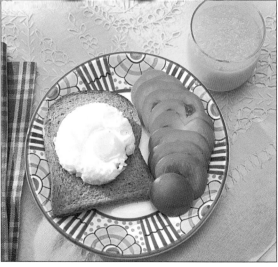

Below left: 2 slices Nimble or Slimcea
bread topped with baked beans and
tomatoes

Below right: Poached egg on toast
with sliced tomato plus orange juice

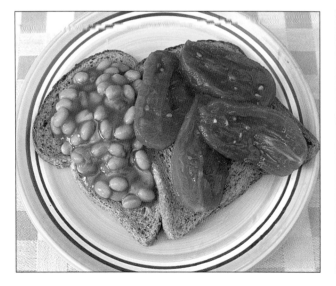

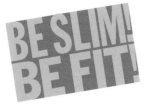

Lunches

SELECT ANY ONE

Quick and Easy Lunches

Ryvitas with Marmite
and cottage cheese

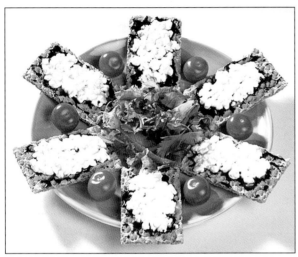

- Heinz Lunch Bowl, plus 1 piece fresh fruit.
- Golden Wonder Pot Light, plus 1 Mullerlight yogurt.
- 4 brown Ryvitas topped with low-fat coleslaw and tomatoes, plus 1 chicken drumstick (no skin).
- Batchelor's Cup a Soup, plus 5 oz (125 g) diet yogurt and 2 pieces fresh fruit (e.g. 4 oz/ 100 g grapes, 4 oz/100 g strawberries).
- 6 brown Ryvitas spread with Marmite and topped with 4 oz (100 g) cottage cheese plus unlimited salad.
- 4 brown Ryvitas spread with horseradish sauce and topped with $2^1/_2$ oz (62.5 g) mackerel fillets in spicy tomato sauce, plus 2 pieces fresh fruit.
- 2 slices Nimble or Slimcea topped with 8 oz (200 g) canned spaghetti hoops, plus 1 apple.
- $^1/_2$ pint (250 ml) clear soup, 2 oz (50 g) wholemeal roll, 2 tomatoes, 4 oz (100 g) cherries.
- 1 chicken leg (no skin) with chopped salad and 1 tablespoon fat-free salad dressing.
- 4 oz (100 g) red kidney beans, 4 oz (100 g) sweetcorn, chopped cucumber, tomatoes, onions, tossed in natural yogurt mixed with mint sauce.
- 2 oz (50 g) ham, 2 oz cottage cheese and mixed salad with fat-free salad dressing.

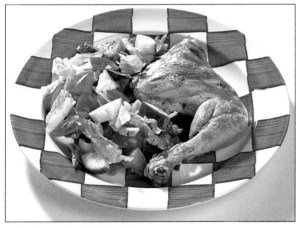

Chicken leg with
chopped salad

- Mix 2 oz (50 g) cooked peas, 2 oz (50 g) canned kidney beans, 2 chopped spring onions or 1 red pepper, deseeded and chopped, with 2 oz (50 g) cooked brown rice and low-fat salad dressing. Top with 2 oz (50 g) cottage cheese.
- 2 oz (50 g) French bread, 2 teaspoons Branston pickle, 2 oz (50 g) wafer-thin beef or pastrami, plus salad.

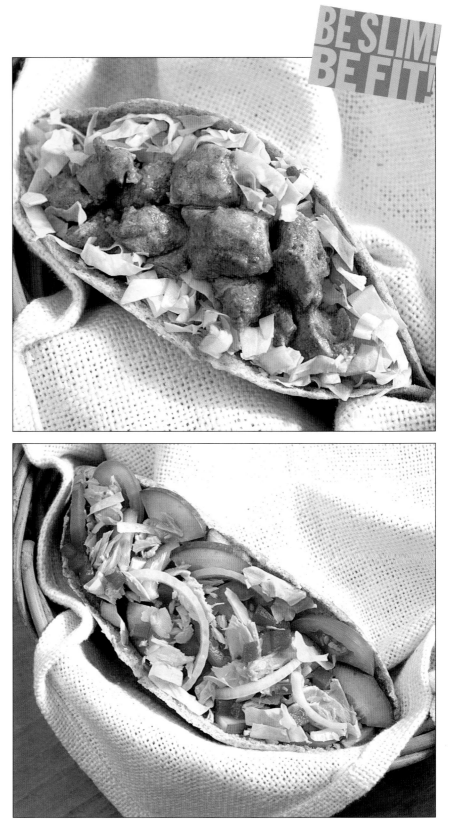

- 2 slices wholemeal bread spread with fat-free salad dressing and filled with 2 oz (50 g) cold, cooked chicken plus salad.
- 2 slices wholemeal bread spread with horseradish sauce and filled with 1 oz (25 g) lean beef and salad.
- Chicken Tikka Pitta: Split open 1 wholemeal pitta bread. Spread the inside with natural yogurt mixed with a little mint sauce. Fill with 3 oz (75 g) chicken tikka (ready prepared or home-made) and shredded salad.
- Tuna or Salmon Pitta: Split open 1 wholemeal pitta bread and filled with 2 oz (50 g) tuna (in brine) or salmon, plus shredded lettuce, sliced tomato, cucumber, onion and pepper.

Above right: Chicken Tikka Pitta
Right: Tuna or Salmon Pitt

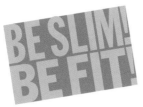

Sandwich Specials

- Ham and Kiwi Open Sandwich: Halve a 5 in (12.5 cm) French stick and spread with fat-free salad dressing and mustard. Top with 2 oz (50 g) lean ham and sliced kiwi fruit.
- Chicken and Salad Roll: Slit one large, long bread roll twice along the top and spread with fat-free salad dressing. Fill with 2 oz (50 g) chicken plus salad.
- Tuna and Salad Sandwich: Spread 2 slices wholemeal bread with horseradish sauce and fill with 2 oz (50 g) tuna (in brine) and lots of salad.
- Cottage Cheese and Pineapple Bap: 2 oz (50 g) bap spread with pineapple jam and filled with 2 oz (50 g) cottage cheese and 3 oz (75 g) fresh pineapple.

Club Sandwich

SERVES 1

2 oz (50 g) uncooked lean bacon
3 slices bread
1 teaspoon reduced-oil salad dressing (any brand)
1 teaspoon tomato ketchup
$\frac{1}{2}$ teaspoon mustard
1 oz (25 g) cooked chicken
1 tomato
Shredded lettuce leaves
4 cocktail sticks

Grill the bacon until well cooked and crisp. Toast the bread and spread one slice with reduced-oil salad dressing, the second slice with tomato ketchup and the third with mustard.

Slice the chicken and tomato and place on the first slice of toast. Next, add the toast spread with tomato ketchup, then add the bacon followed by shredded lettuce. Top with the remaining piece of toast (spread with mustard). Press together firmly. Cut into 4 triangles crossways and pierce each quarter segment with a cocktail stick to secure.

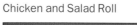

Ham and Kiwi Open Sandwich

Chicken and Salad Roll

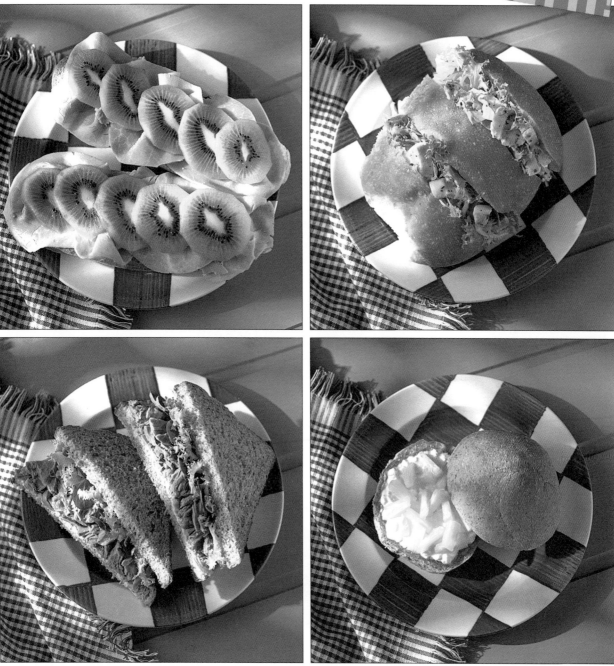

Tuna and Salad Sandwich

Cottage Cheese and Pineapple Bap

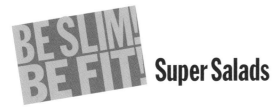

Super Salads

Rice Salad

SERVES 1

1 green pepper, deseeded
1 tomato
2 in (5 cm) cucumber
2 oz (50 g) (dry weight) rice,
boiled, rinsed and drained
1 oz (25 g) peas, cooked
1 oz (25 g) sweetcorn, cooked
Soy sauce
Salt and black pepper

Chop the pepper, tomato and cucumber very finely and mix in with the rice, peas and sweetcorn. Add soy sauce and seasoning to taste.

Courgette and Tomato Salad

SERVES 4

2 small heads chicory
4 tomatoes
2 courgettes
1 bunch radishes
5 oz (125 g) fromage frais or yogurt
$\frac{1}{2}$ teaspoon French mustard
1 tablespoon chopped gherkin *or* 1 tablespoon chopped spring onions
1 tablespoon chopped fresh parsley
Salt and black pepper

Wash the chicory. Reserve a few leaves for garnishing and slice the rest. Skin and seed the tomatoes and chop the flesh coarsely. Trim the courgettes, cut into 2–3 pieces, slice lengthways, then cut into matchstick-sized pieces. Coarsely grate half the radishes and slice the remainder. Mix together the fromage frais or yogurt, mustard, gherkins or spring onions, and parsley and season to taste.

Mix the sliced chicory, tomatoes, courgettes and grated radishes together. Fold in the sauce and pile the salad on to a dish.

Garnish each end of the dish with the reserved leaves of chicory. Arrange the sliced radishes down the side of the dish.

Chill until required.

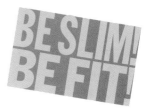

Chinese and Apple Salad

SERVES 2

1 red apple
1 green apple
A few radishes
2 sticks celery
A few spring onions
1 tablespoon lemon juice
6 oz (150 g) beansprouts
Curly lettuce to decorate

For the sweet 'n' sour dressing
$1\frac{1}{2}$ tablespoons lemon juice
1 level tablespoon clear honey
A few drops soy sauce

Slice both apples and remove the cores. Slice the radishes, celery and spring onions.

Mix the apples and lemon juice thoroughly, then add the beansprouts, radishes, celery and spring onions.

Place all the dressing ingredients into a screw-top jar and shake well. Pour the dressing over the salad and toss well. Decorate with the lettuce and serve immediately.

Below left: Courgette and Tomato Salad
Below right: Chinese and Apple Salad

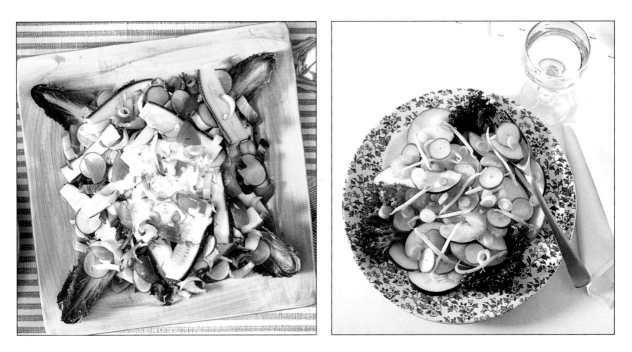

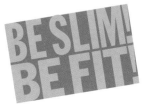

Inch Loss Salad

SERVES 1

Unlimited amounts of shredded lettuce, chopped cucumber and other
green salad items
1 apple, peeled, cored and sliced
1 kiwi fruit, peeled and sliced
1 orange, peeled and cut into segments
1 pear, peeled, cored and sliced
2 oz (50 g) chopped, cooked chicken *or* cooked, shelled prawns

For the dressing
1 tablespoon wine vinegar
2 tablespoons natural yogurt
1 clove garlic, crushed
Salt and black pepper to taste

Place the lettuce and green salad on a large dinner plate. Arrange the
various fruits around the edge of the salad, and place the chicken or
prawns in the centre.

Mix the dressing ingredients together and serve with the salad.

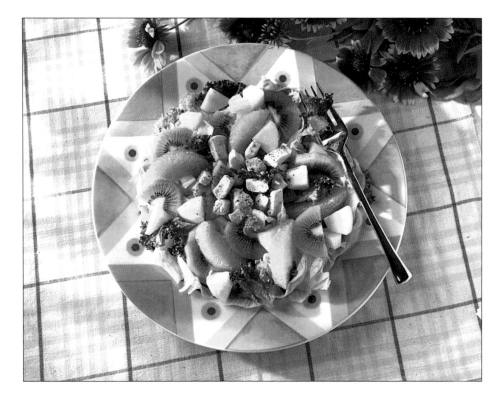

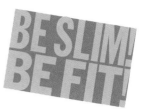

Soups

- 16 oz (400 g) can Heinz Vegetable Soup and 1 oz (25 g) French bread (no butter).
- 16 oz (400 g) can Baxters Cock-a-Leekie Soup plus 2 brown Ryvitas spread with Marmite.
- 16 oz (400 g) can Baxters Scotch Broth plus 2 pieces fresh fruit.
- 16 oz (400 g) can Baxters Mediterranean Soup plus 1 slice wholemeal toast (no butter) and 5 oz (125 g) diet yogurt.
- 1 can Crosse & Blackwell Condensed Vegetable Soup, reconstituted, plus 1 slice wholemeal bread (no butter).
- 1 can Crosse & Blackwell Condensed Mushroom Soup, reconstituted, plus 1 slice wholemeal bread (no butter).
- 1 can Weight Watchers Chicken Soup plus 1 slice wholemeal toast (no butter) and 1 banana.
- 16 oz (400 g) can potato and leek soup plus 1 slice wholemeal toast (no butter) and 4 oz (100 g) grapes.
- 16 oz (400 g) can Heinz Oxtail Soup plus 1 slice wholemeal bread (no butter).

Tomato and Lentil Soup

SERVES 4

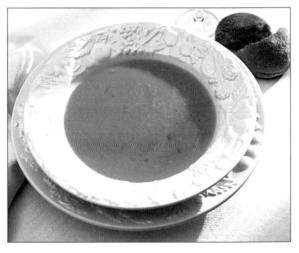

3 cloves garlic, peeled and crushed
1 medium onion, peeled and chopped
1$\frac{1}{2}$ pints (750 ml) vegetable stock
6 tomatoes, skinned and chopped
8 oz (200 g) carrots, roughly grated
8 oz (200 g) potatoes, peeled and diced
4 oz (100 g) split red lentils, presoaked
Salt and pepper to taste

In a non-stick frying pan dry-fry the garlic and onion until soft. Add $\frac{1}{4}$ pint (125 ml) of the vegetable stock.

Stir in the tomatoes, carrots, potatoes and lentils. Cover and cook for 10 minutes, stirring occasionally to prevent the mixture from burning.

Pour in the remaining stock and add the seasoning. Bring to the boil then simmer gently for 30 minutes.

Sieve or liquidise the soup. Check the seasoning and reheat. Serve piping hot with 1 slice wholemeal bread per person.

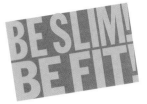

Creamy Vegetable Soup

SERVES 4

$1\frac{1}{4}$ lb (500 g) potatoes, peeled and diced
8 oz (200 g) carrots, trimmed, scraped and sliced
$2\frac{1}{2}$ pints (1.5 litres) vegetable stock
2 oz (50 g) skimmed milk powder (in addition to allowance)
1 oz (25 g) cornflour
Chopped fresh parsley to garnish

Place all the vegetables in a saucepan with the vegetable stock. Season, cover and simmer for 20–30 minutes.

Blend the skimmed milk powder and cornflour with a little cold water and stir into the soup. Bring to the boil and simmer for 5 minutes, stirring continuously.

Garnish with the parsley and serve with 1 slice wholemeal bread per person.

Tomato and Orange Soup

SERVES 4

1 large onion, peeled and grated
1 large carrot, trimmed, scraped and grated
1 x 14 oz (350 g) can chopped tomatoes
8 oz (200 g) potatoes, peeled and thinly sliced
1 teaspoon mixed herbs
$\frac{1}{2}$ teaspoon demerara sugar
Zest and juice of 1 orange
1 pint (500 ml) chicken stock
Salt and black pepper to taste
5 oz (125 g) natural yogurt
Parsley sprigs to garnish

In a non-stick saucepan gently dry-fry the onion for 5 minutes then add the grated carrots and cook for a further 2 minutes.

Add the remaining ingredients, except the yogurt, and simmer gently for 30 minutes.

Liquidise the soup in a blender, or pass through a sieve. Add the yogurt, adjust the seasoning and reheat, but do not boil.

Garnish with the parsley sprigs and serve with 1 slice wholemeal bread per person.

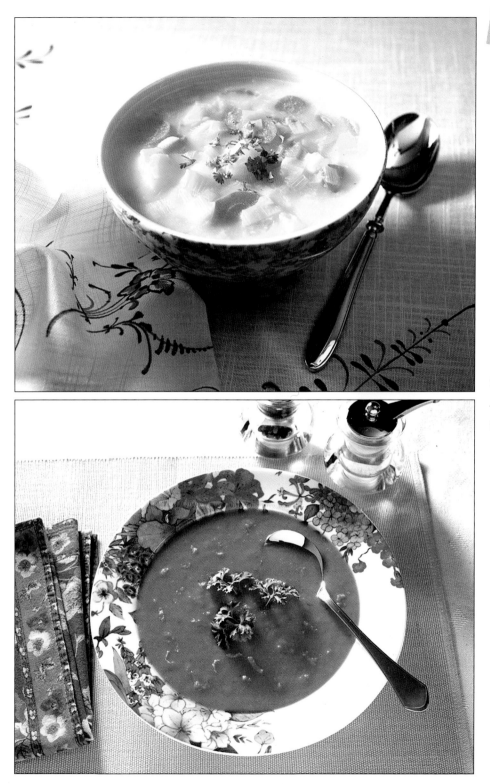

Creamy Vegetable Soup

Tomato and Orange
Soup

THE BE SLIM! BE FIT! EATING PLAN   53

Jacket Potato Lunches

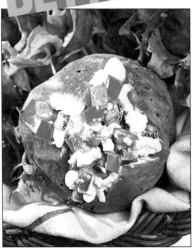

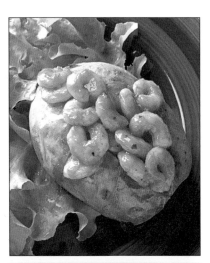

- 8 oz (200 g) jacket potato topped with 4 oz (100 g) cottage cheese mixed with 3 oz (75 g) chopped green and red peppers plus salad.

- 8 oz (200 g) jacket potato topped with 2 oz (50 g) prawns in 2 tablespoons reduced-oil salad dressing mixed with 2 tablespoons tomato ketchup, plus salad.

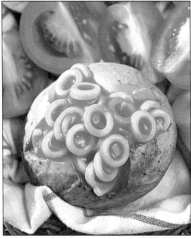

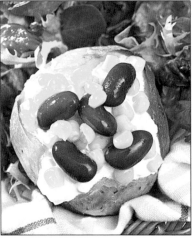

- 8 oz (200 g) jacket potato topped with 8 oz (200 g) canned spaghetti hoops or baked beans, plus 2 tomatoes.

- 8 oz (200 g) jacket potato topped with 2 oz (50 g) cottage cheese mixed with 1 oz (25 g) red kidney beans and 1 oz (25 g) sweetcorn, plus salad.

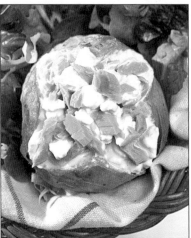

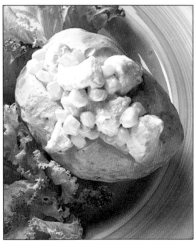

- 8 oz (200 g) jacket potato topped with 2 oz (50 g) cottage cheese mixed with 2 oz (50 g) canned salmon or tuna (in brine) and 1 tablespoon low-fat salad dressing, plus salad.

- 8 oz (200 g) jacket potato topped with 1 oz (25 g) diced chicken, 2 oz (50 g) sweetcorn mixed with natural yogurt, plus salad.

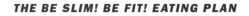

Chilli Bacon Potato

SERVES 1

1 medium-sized potato
2 oz (50 g) lean bacon, chopped
1 small onion, peeled and chopped
4 mushrooms, washed and chopped
2 tablespoons chilli sauce

Bake the potato in the oven or microwave.
Dry-fry the bacon, onion and mushrooms in a non-stick frying pan. When cooked, add the chilli sauce and mix well.
Remove the cooked potato from the oven or microwave, slice it in half lengthways and top with the chilli bacon mixture. Serve immediately.

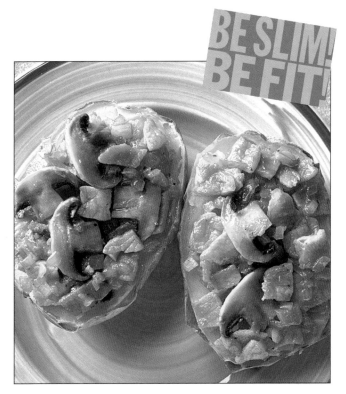

Ratatouille Potatoes

SERVES 4

4 x 8 oz (4 x 200 g) potatoes
1 medium onion, peeled and thinly sliced
1 small aubergine, finely sliced
2 courgettes, thinly sliced
1 red or green pepper, deseeded and sliced
$7\frac{1}{2}$ oz (187.5 g) can chopped tomatoes
1 clove garlic, peeled and crushed
Salt and black pepper

Bake the potatoes in the oven or microwave.
Dry-fry the onions in a non-stick frying pan until soft but not brown. Add the remaining ingredients, bring to the boil and simmer for 20–25 minutes.
When the potatoes are cooked, cut each in half lengthways and fill with the ratatouille mixture. Serve immediately.

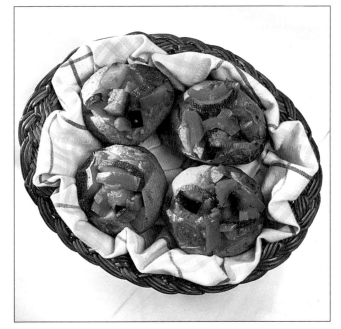

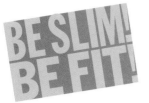

Dinners

SELECT ANY STARTER,
MAIN COURSE AND DESSERT

Starters

- Prawn Cocktail: Use 3 oz (75 g) prawns per person. Serve on a bed of lettuce with low-calorie salad dressing mixed with tomato ketchup (half and half).
- 8 oz (200 g) canned grapefruit in natural juice.
- Chopped melon mixed with 2 oz (50g) seedless grapes.
- Carrot and Banana Cocktail: 1 grated carrot mixed with $\frac{1}{2}$ banana, sliced, and 10 sultanas. Sprinkle with lemon juice.
- Mixed salad with dressing of 3 oz (75 g) natural yogurt with 1 teaspoon mint sauce.
- 4 oz (100 g) melon with 4 oz (100 g) strawberries.
- 1 oz (25 g) parma ham with fan of melon.
- 1 corn on the cob (frozen or tinned).
- Kiwi and Melon Salad: Mix together cubes of melon (use a selection of different types of melon for added colour) with peeled and sliced kiwi fruit.
- Melon and Mango Salad: Peel and deseed a wedge of melon. Slice it but don't cut right through the flesh. Peel a mango and cut a large piece from the centre 'stone'. Slice in the same way as the melon. Serve the melon and mango together on a plate, and garnish with strawberries.
- Pair of Pears: Take a ripe pear. Peel, halve lengthways and remove the core, and paint with lemon juice to prevent discolouration. Fill the cavities with cottage cheese and serve on shredded lettuce.
- Crudités: Serve assorted raw vegetable sticks (carrots, peppers, celery, cucumber) with a dip of natural yogurt mixed with a little mint sauce.

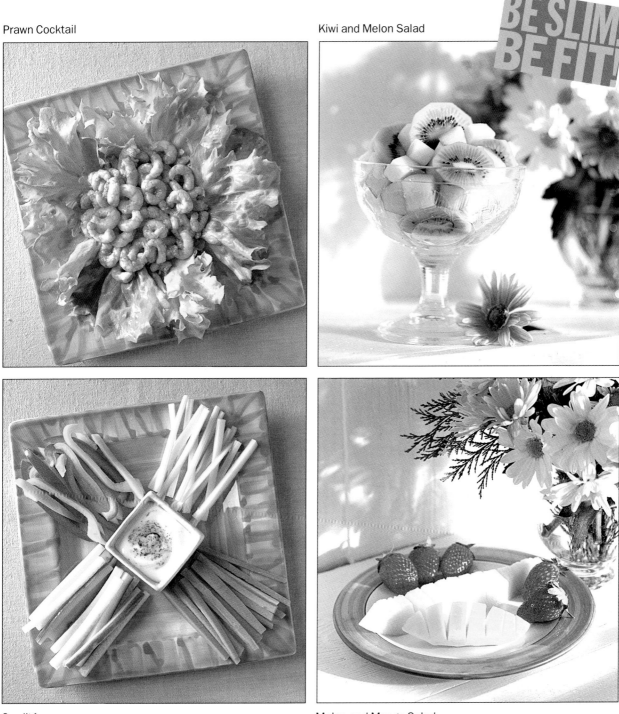

Prawn Cocktail

Kiwi and Melon Salad

Crudités

Melon and Mango Salad

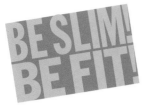

Waldorf Salad

SERVES 4

1 head of celery
2 apples
6 oz (150 g) canned water chestnuts
2 tablespoons lemon juice
2 oz (50 g) sultanas
5 oz (125 g) natural yogurt
3 tablespoons reduced-oil salad dressing
Salt and pepper to taste

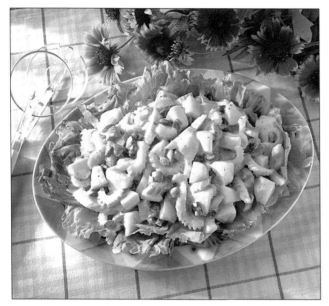

Core and chop the apples. Wash and chop the water chestnuts and mix together with the lemon juice and apples.

Mix all the remaining ingredients in a bowl and pour over the salad. Stir well to ensure a thorough coating. Keep chilled until ready to serve.

Serve on a bed of lettuce within two hours of preparation.

Melon and Prawn Salad

SERVES 1

1 melon
4 oz (100 g) prawns, shelled

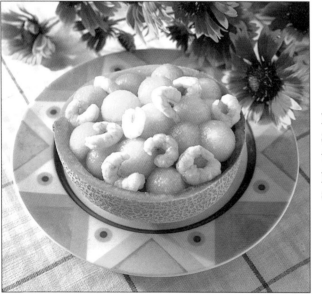

Halve the melon and remove the seeds. Scoop out the flesh with a ball-scoop. Mix the melon balls carefully with the shelled prawns and place in the empty melon shells.

Serve chilled.

Grilled Grapefruit

SERVES 2

1 grapefruit
2 tablespoons sweet sherry
2 teaspoons demerara sugar
2 tablespoons fromage frais

Cut the grapefruit in half. Using a grapefruit knife, remove the core and membranes between segments. Pour the sherry over the flesh, and sprinkle the sugar over. Place in a heatproof dish and then place under a hot grill until the sugar is glazed.

Serve hot, topped with fromage frais.

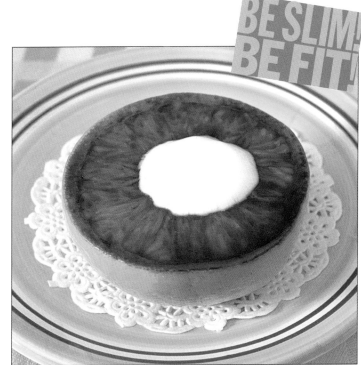

Orange and Grapefruit Cocktail

SERVES 2

1 large orange
1 grapefruit

Remove the peel and pith from both fruits. Work the segments from the core with a sharp knife and arrange in two dishes. Squeeze as much juice as possible from the peel and core on to the fruit.

Serve chilled.

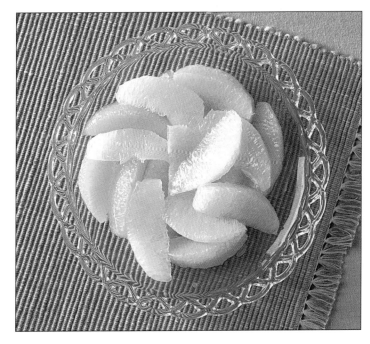

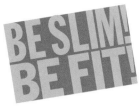

Regular Main Courses

Below: Roast beef with Dry-roast Potatoes; carrots, Brussels sprouts, peas, French beans and gravy

Foot: Roast pork with Dry-roast Potatoes; Brussels sprouts, carrots, cauliflower and gravy

- 4 oz (100 g) roast beef, served with Dry-roast Potatoes (see recipe), boiled carrots, Brussels sprouts, peas and French beans served without butter, plus gravy made without fat.
- 5 oz (125 g) roast pork served with unlimited Dry-roast Potatoes (see recipe), Brussels sprouts, carrots, cauliflower and fat-free gravy.
- 6 oz (150 g) chopped chicken, stir-fried in soy sauce with onions and mushrooms and served on a bed of boiled rice (2 oz/50 g dry weight).
- 4 oz (100 g) fillet steak grilled, topped with green peppercorns in fromage frais and served with 6 oz (150 g) jacket potato topped with fromage frais and chives, plus peas, tomatoes and mushrooms.
- Pork chop (6 oz/150 g cooked weight including bone), grilled with all fat removed, served with 2 oz (50 g) apple sauce, 2 oz (50 g) sage and onion stuffing, plus new potatoes, carrots, chopped cabbage, sweetcorn kernels and fat-free gravy.
- 3 lamb chops (8 oz/200 g total cooked weight including bone) grilled with all fat removed and served with mint sauce, parsnips, carrots, peas and potatoes creamed with natural yogurt.

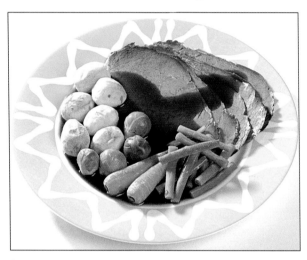

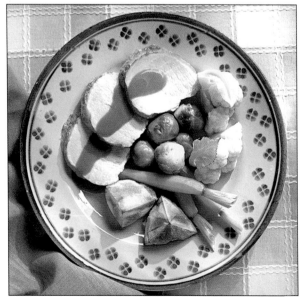

Dry-roast Potatoes

1 lb (400 g) medium-sized potatoes
1 vegetable stock cube

Peel the potatoes and place in a saucepan of boiling water with the stock cube. Cook for 5 minutes.

Remove the potatoes from the saucepan with a slotted spoon and place on a baking tray.

Cook in a moderate oven (200°C, 400°F, or Gas Mark 6) for about one hour or until brown and crisp.

Fillet steak with green peppercorns in fromage frais; jacket potato topped with fromage frais and chives; peas, tomatoes and mushrooms

Chopped chicken in soy sauce with onions, mushrooms and rice

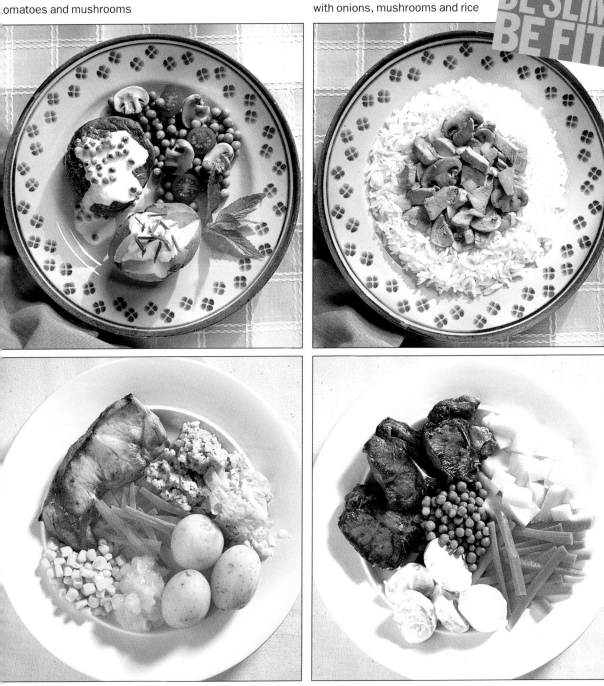

Pork chop with apple sauce and sage and onion stuffing; new potatoes, carrots, cabbage, sweetcorn and gravy

Lamb chops with mint sauce; potatoes creamed with yogurt; parsnips, carrots, peas

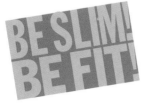

Shepherd's Pie

SERVES 4

1 lb (400 g) lean minced beef
$^1/_2$ pint (250 ml) water
1 large onion, peeled and finely chopped
1 teaspoon mixed herbs
1 teaspoon yeast or beef and vegetable extract
1 teaspoon gravy powder
$1^1/_2$ lb (600 g) potatoes, peeled
Salt and black pepper

Boil the mince in the water in a saucepan for five minutes. Drain the mince and place in a covered container until required. Place the drained liquid in a bowl in the refrigerator (this will cause any fat to rise to the top and set hard so that it can be discarded).

Return the skimmed liquid to the saucepan. Add the mince, onion, herbs and the yeast or beef and vegetable extract. Mix the gravy powder with a little water and add to the meat mixture. Bring to the boil, stirring continuously, and leave to simmer for a further 10 minutes.

Boil the potatoes until soft, then remove most, but not all, of the water. Mash the potatoes and season well, adding a little skimmed or semi-skimmed milk, if necessary, to make a soft consistency.

Place the mince mixture in an ovenproof dish and cover with the mashed potatoes. Place under a preheated grill to brown the top, or place in a preheated oven (160°C, 325°F, or Gas Mark 3) for 10 minutes.

Serve with unlimited vegetables.

Liver and Onion Casserole

SERVES 4

2 large onions
1 lb (400 g) lambs' liver
$^3/_4$ pint (375 ml) vegetable stock
Salt and black pepper to taste
1 level tablespoon gravy powder

Peel and slice the onions. Preheat a non-stick pan and dry-fry the onions until soft and brown.

Slice the liver and add to the pan. Add the vegetable stock and cook thoroughly. Thicken with gravy powder mixed with water.

Serve with potatoes, carrots and cabbage.

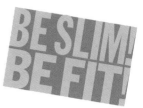

Soufflé Potato and Ham Bake

SERVES 4

8 oz (200 g) broccoli, cut into spears
and blanched
1¼ lb (500 g) potatoes, peeled
and cooked
2 tablespoons skimmed or semi-
skimmed milk (in addition to
allowance)
1 tablespoon natural yogurt
1 oz (25 g) plain flour
Salt and black pepper to taste
3 eggs, separated
6 spring onions, chopped
6 oz (150 g) smoked ham, chopped
1 tablespoon fresh chives, chopped
½ teaspoon paprika

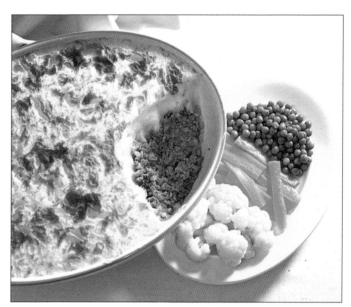

Shepherd's Pie with vegetables

Place the broccoli in the base of a
lightly greased, 7 inch (18 cm) soufflé
dish.

Mash the potatoes with the milk and
yogurt. Work in the flour and season
well. Stir in the egg yolks, spring
onions, ham and chives.

Whisk the egg whites until they
form soft peaks, then gently but
thoroughly fold into the potato mixture.

Spread the mixture on top of the
broccoli and sprinkle with paprika.
Bake in a preheated oven at 200°C, 400°F,
or Gas Mark 6 for 25 minutes or until
well risen and golden brown.

Serve immediately with fresh
vegetables.

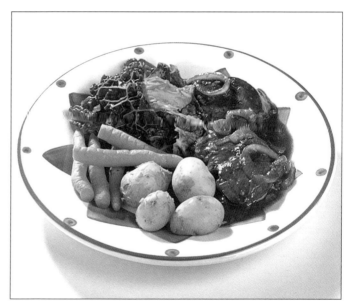

Liver and Onion Casserole with vegetables

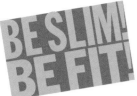

Quick and Easy Main Courses

- 4 grilled fish fingers served with tomato sauce and 6 oz (150 g) potatoes mashed with yogurt, plus peas and carrots.
- 1 pack Bird's Eye Chicken with Gravy (serves 1), served with potatoes, cauliflower, broccoli and peas.
- 6 oz (150 g) chicken breast (no skin) chopped and dry-fried with Uncle Ben's Stir-fry Sauce and served with 2 oz/50 g (dry weight) boiled brown rice.
- Chicken Provençale (serves 4): Chop 1 lb (400 g) chicken breast and dry-fry with 1 chopped onion. When almost cooked, add 1 jar Uncle Ben's Provençale with Peppers and Onion Sauce and cook for 5 minutes. Serve with boiled brown rice (2 oz/50 g dry weight per person).
- Coq au Vin (serves 4): Place 4 x 6 oz (4 x 150 g) chicken breasts, 2 sliced onions and 4 oz (100 g) sliced mushrooms in an ovenproof dish. Add contents of 1 sachet Colman's Coq au Vin Casserole Mix mixed with $^{3}/_{4}$ pint (375 ml) water and stir well. Cover and cook in a preheated oven for $1^{1}/_{2}$ hours at 180°C, 350°F, or Gas Mark 4. Serve with unlimited vegetables.
- Chinese Chicken with Pineapple Sauce (serves 4): Chop $1^{1}/_{2}$ lb (600 g) chicken breasts into bite-sized pieces and dry-fry in a non-stick pan. Add 1 jar of Del Monte Quality Chinese with Pineapple Sauce. Serve with boiled brown rice (2 oz/50 g dry weight per person).
- Chicken Chasseur (serves 4): Place 4 chicken breasts, 1 sliced onion and 4 oz (100 g) button mushrooms in a casserole dish. Add 1 can Homepride Chicken Chasseur Cook-in-Sauce and cook according to instructions. Serve with unlimited vegetables.
- Chicken in Black Bean Sauce (serves 4): Chop 1 lb (400 g) chicken breasts into bite-sized pieces and dry-fry with 1 chopped onion in a non-stick pan. Add 1 jar Uncle Ben's Black Bean Sauce. Serve with boiled brown rice (2 oz/50 g dry weight per person).
- Chicken in Basil and Chilli Sauce (serves 4): Chop $1^{1}/_{2}$ lb (600 g) chicken breasts into bite-sized pieces and dry-fry with 2 chopped red peppers and $^{1}/_{2}$ can bamboo shoots. Add 6 oz (150 g) jar Sharwood's Basil and Chilli Sauce. Serve with boiled brown rice.
- Pork Casserole (serves 4): Chop 1 lb (400 g) lean pork, 2 peeled onions, 2 large carrots and 4 oz (100 g) green beans. Place in a casserole dish with 1 sachet Coleman's Traditional Pork Casserole Mix mixed with

Fish fingers with potatoes creamed with yogurt; peas, carrots and tomato sauce

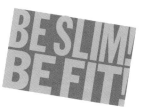

³/₄ pint (375 ml) water and stir well. Cover and cook in a preheated oven for 1¹/₂ hours at 180°C, 350°F, or Gas Mark 4 until the pork is tender. Serve with unlimited vegetables and potatoes.

- Spicy Sweet and Sour Pork (serves 2): Chop 12 oz (300 g) pork and dry-fry with 1 chopped onion. When almost cooked, add contents of 14¹/₂ oz (360 g) jar Uncle Ben's Extra Spicy Stir-fry Sweet and Sour Sauce with Crispy Vegetables. Serve with unlimited vegetables and boiled rice (2 oz/50 g dry weight per person).
- Findus Lean Cuisine Prawn Curry with Rice.
- 299 g can (serves 2) Prince's Stewed Steak with Gravy, served with unlimited vegetables.

Coq au Vin with vegetables · Spicy Sweet and Sour Pork with rice

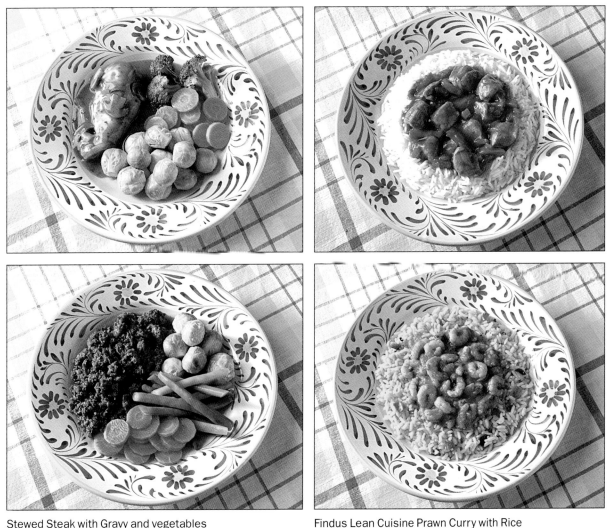

Stewed Steak with Gravy and vegetables · Findus Lean Cuisine Prawn Curry with Rice

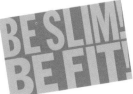

Chicken Dishes

Moray Chicken

SERVES 4

4 chicken breasts, skinned and boned
2 medium onions, peeled and chopped
2 sticks celery, diced
2 medium carrots, thinly sliced
1 lb (400 g) potatoes, peeled and cubed
$\frac{1}{4}$ pint (125 ml) white wine
$\frac{1}{4}$ pint (125 ml) chicken stock
Salt and black pepper to taste
1 teaspoon cornflour, blended with a little water
5 oz (125 g) fromage frais
Chopped fresh parsley to garnish

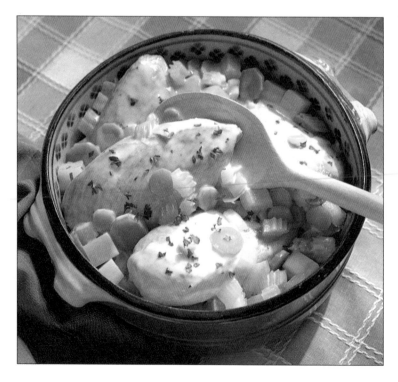

In a non-stick frying pan lightly dry-fry the chicken to seal. Add the vegetables to the pan and sauté for 5 minutes. Pour in the wine and stock and season well. Bring to the boil, cover, and simmer gently for 45 minutes. Using a slotted spoon, remove the chicken and vegetables and place in a serving dish.

Pour the blended cornflour into the pan, stirring continuously. Bring back to the boil and check the seasoning. Blend the fromage frais into the sauce and pour over the chicken.

Garnish with the fresh parsley and serve with fresh green vegetables.

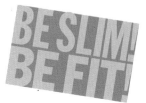

Chicken and Mushroom Bake

SERVES 2

3 medium-sized potatoes
6 oz (150 g) cooked chicken, diced
1 clove garlic, peeled and thinly sliced
1 oz (25 g) frozen peas
2 spring onions, finely chopped
Black pepper to taste
3 oz (75 g) mushrooms, sliced
1 packet Batchelor's Cup a Soup
(Chicken and Sweetcorn or Chicken and Mushroom)

Scrub the potatoes and boil with the skins on until cooked.

Meanwhile, place the chicken in the bottom of an ovenproof casserole dish. Add the garlic, frozen peas and spring onions. Season with black pepper. Lay the mushrooms over the top of the chicken.

In a cup, make up the Cup a Soup a little thicker than usual, removing the croutons. Reserve a quarter of the soup mixture and pour the remainder into the casserole.

Drain and slice the potatoes and lay them over the casserole mixture. Spoon the remaining soup over the potatoes.

Bake uncovered in a preheated oven at 190°C, 375°F, or Gas Mark 5 for 15 minutes.

Serve with unlimited vegetables.

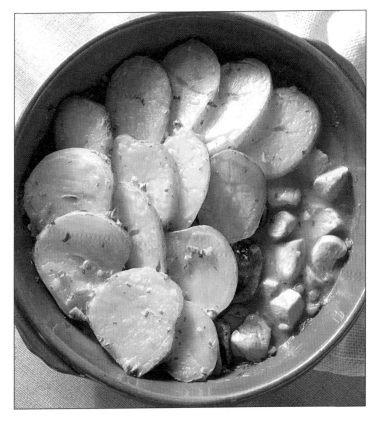

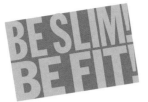

Tarragon Chicken

SERVES 4

4 skinless chicken fillets
1 medium onion, peeled and chopped
12 button mushrooms, halved
1 chicken stock cube dissolved in $\frac{1}{4}$ pint (125 ml) boiling water
3 teaspoons fresh tarragon, chopped
Salt and black pepper to taste
1 tablespoon cornflour
2 tablespoons natural yogurt
2 oz (50 g) seedless grapes

Place the chicken, onion, mushrooms, chicken stock, tarragon and seasoning into a shallow casserole dish. Cover, and cook in a preheated oven at 180°C, 350°F, or Gas Mark 4 for approximately one hour, ensuring that the chicken is cooked thoroughly.

Blend the cornflour with a little water and stir into the casserole mixture. Return the casserole to the oven for 5 minutes and allow to thicken.

Stir in the yogurt and grapes, and serve immediately with potatoes and unlimited vegetables.

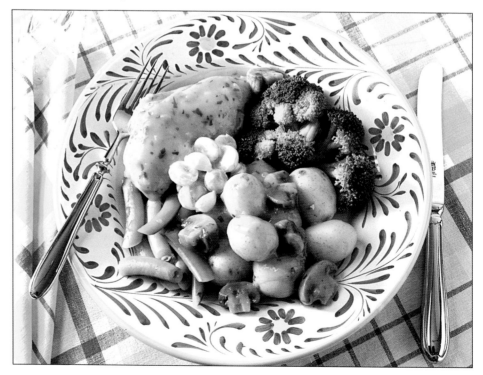

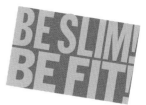

Chilli Chicken

SERVES 2

1 medium onion, peeled and chopped
2 cloves garlic, peeled and crushed
2 fresh green chillies, crushed or finely chopped (including seeds)
8 oz (200 g) chicken breast, chopped (all skin removed)
1 x 8 oz (200 g) can chopped tomatoes
1 teaspoon tomato purée
Good squeeze lemon or lime juice
1 teaspoon dried oregano
Salt and sugar to taste
2 tablespoons fromage frais

Dry-fry the onion, garlic and chillies until softened. If the mixture begins to stick add 1 tablespoon of water. Add the chicken and stir continuously for 4–5 minutes. Stir in the tomatoes, tomato purée, lemon or lime juice and oregano.

Bring to the boil, reduce the heat, then simmer for 20 minutes. Add the salt and sugar to taste. Remove from the heat and stir in the fromage frais.

Serve immediately with boiled rice (2 oz/50 g dry weight per person) and unlimited salad.

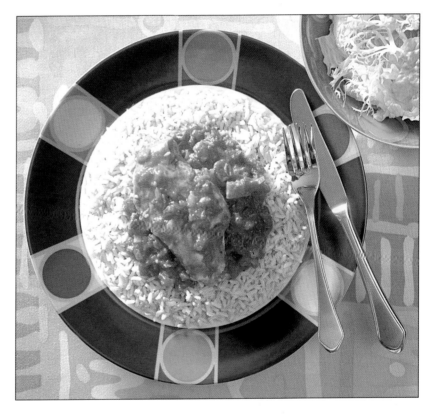

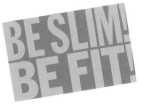

Fish Dishes

Cod with potatoes creamed with yogurt; sweetcorn, carrots, broccoli and tomato sauce

- 8 oz (200 g) cod or haddock, steamed or microwaved without fat, served with potatoes creamed with natural yogurt (no butter), sweetcorn, carrots and broccoli, plus tomato sauce.
- 1 trout, microwaved, served with unlimited vegetables and potatoes. Garnish with lemon.

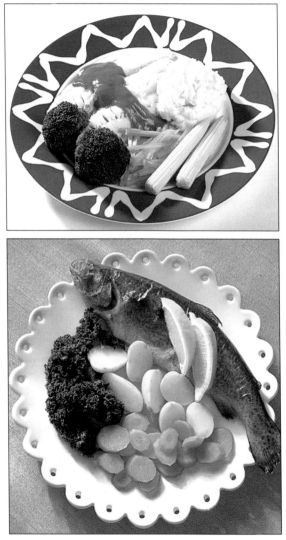

Trout with vegetables and potatoes

Cod in Parsley Sauce

SERVES 1

6 oz (150 g) cod
2 teaspoons cornflour
$1/4$ pint (125 ml) skimmed or semi-skimmed milk
(in addition to allowance)
Chopped fresh parsley to taste

Place the cod in a little of the milk in a saucepan. Cover and simmer gently for 10–15 minutes. Drain.

In a saucepan blend the cornflour with a little of the remaining milk to form a smooth paste. Heat gently, adding the remaining milk and stirring continuously.

Just before serving add the parsley. Serve the fish, topped with the sauce, with unlimited vegetables and potatoes.

Fish Pie

SERVES 4

$1^{1}/_{2}$ lb (600 g) cod
$1^{1}/_{2}$ lb (600 g) potatoes
Salt and black pepper to taste

Bake, steam or microwave the fish, but do not overcook.

Boil the potatoes until well done and mash with a little water to make a soft consistency. Season well.

Place the fish in an ovenproof dish. Flake the flesh, remove the skin, and distribute the fish evenly across the base of the dish. Season well.

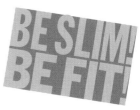

Cover the fish completely with the mashed potatoes and smooth over with a fork.

If the ingredients are still hot, just place under a hot grill for a few minutes to brown the top. Alternatively, the pie can be made in advance and then warmed through in a preheated oven at 180°C, 350°F, or Gas Mark 4 for 20 minutes, or microwaved on high for 5 minutes.

Serve with unlimited broccoli, sweetcorn and carrots, plus tomato sauce.

Prawn Stir-fry

SERVES 4

6 sticks celery
3 carrots
1 medium onion
15 oz (375 g) canned beansprouts or
8 oz (200 g) fresh beansprouts
16 oz (400 g) shelled prawns
Soy sauce
Black pepper

Wash and chop the celery. Peel the carrots and onion and coarsely grate both. If using canned beansprouts, drain well. Place all the ingredients in a wok or non-stick frying pan and cook carefully, tossing them regularly to avoid burning. The juices from the vegetables should prevent them from sticking to the pan. Ensure the prawns are thoroughly cooked.

Serve with boiled brown rice (2 oz/50 g dry weight per person) and extra soy sauce.

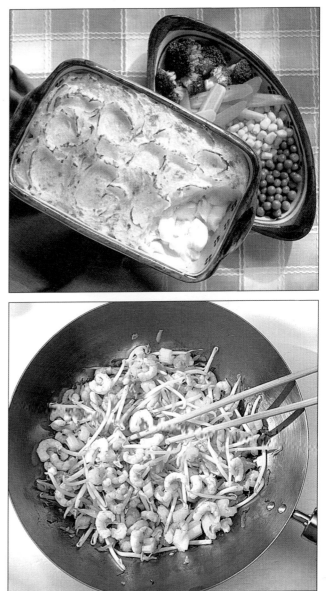

Fish Pie with broccoli, sweetcorn and carrots

Prawn Stir-fry

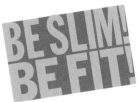

Barbecue Specials

- Barbecued Lamb Kebabs: Cut lean lamb (4 oz/100 g per person) into cubes. Chop green and red peppers and a Spanish onion into bite-size pieces. Thread alternately on to skewers together with button mushrooms and coat with fat-free barbecue sauce. Cook on a hot barbecue, turning regularly. Serve with low-fat coleslaw.

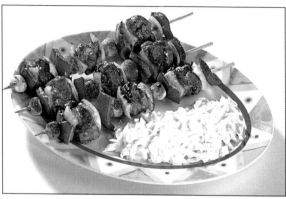

- Barbecued Chicken Drumsticks: Allow 2 drumsticks per person. Paint skinned chicken drumsticks in fat-free barbecue sauce and cook thoroughly on a hot barbecue. Serve with a chopped salad.
- Bacon and Potato Rolls: Par-boil new potatoes and wrap a rasher of lean bacon around each one. Carefully secure with a cocktail stick and cook on a moderate heat on a barbecue. Serve with grated raw carrot mixed with sultanas.

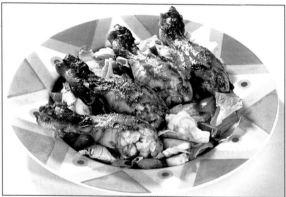

Hamburgers

SERVES 4

1 onion, peeled and chopped
1 lb (400 g) lean minced beef
3 tablespoons breadcrumbs
4 tablespoons skimmed or
semi-skimmed milk
4 burger buns
4 tomato slices
Tomato ketchup

Mix the chopped onion, minced beef, breadcrumbs and milk in a large bowl. Leave for 10 minutes and then make up the mixture into 4 hamburgers. Cook on a hot barbecue for 5 minutes each side. Place each burger in a bun with a slice of tomato and tomato ketchup.

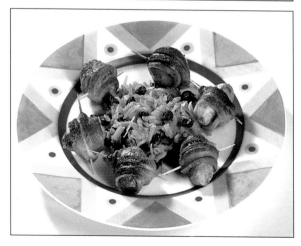

From top to bottom:
Barbecued Lamb Kebabs with coleslaw
Barbecued Chicken Drumsticks with salad
Bacon and Potato Rolls with sultanas and grated carrot

Beef or Pork Kebabs

SERVES 4

1 lb (400 g) lean beef or boneless pork
Barbecue sauce (any low-fat brand)
1 large onion
1 red pepper
1 green pepper
2 courgettes
Mushrooms (optional)
12 cherry tomatoes
4 long (or 8 short) skewers
8 oz (200 g) (dry weight) rice, boiled
1 x 16 oz (1 x 400 g) can beansprouts

Cut the beef or pork into one-inch (2.5 cm) cubes and marinate in the barbecue sauce for at least one hour, preferably two, before cooking.

Prepare the vegetables by peeling the onion and cutting into squares. Slice the courgettes thickly and trim the mushrooms, if used. Any remaining vegetables can be cooked and served separately.

Thread the vegetables and beef or pork alternately on to the hot skewers until all the ingredients have been used up or the skewers are full.

Brush the kebabs with the remaining barbecue sauce and cook thoroughly on a hot barbecue, turning them frequently to prevent burning.

When the kebabs are thoroughly cooked, serve on a bed of boiled rice mixed with beansprouts. Heat any remaining sauce and serve with the kebabs.

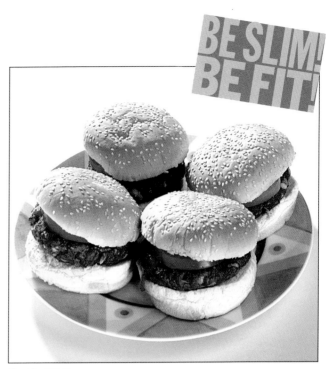

Hamburgers

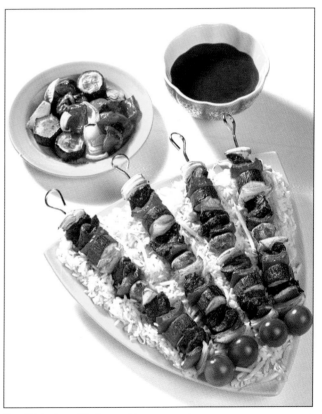

Beef Kebabs with rice and beansprouts

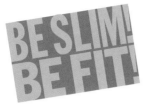

American Turkey Burgers

SERVES 4

3 level tablespoons dry sage and onion stuffing
12 tablespoons boiling water
12 oz (300 g) fresh turkey mince
1 egg white
$\frac{1}{2}$ medium onion, peeled and chopped
Salt and black pepper to taste
4 x 2 oz (4 x 50 g) burger buns

In a large bowl stir the stuffing mix into the water and leave to stand for one minute.

Add the turkey, egg white and onion, and season to taste.

Mix well and, using your hands, divide the mixture into 8 balls and press into burger shapes (or use a burger press). Place on a plate and leave to chill in the refrigerator for at least 15 minutes.

Remove from the refrigerator and cook on a hot barbecue, turning frequently. Ensure the burgers are cooked throughout.

Serve in the burger buns with unlimited salad, tomatoes and relish.

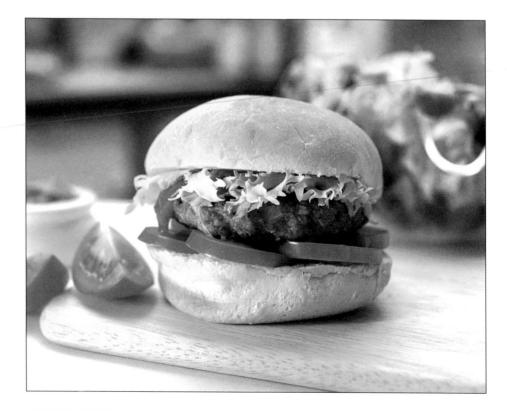

Pasta Dishes

- Chicken in Black Bean Sauce: Use 4 oz (100 g) chicken per person and stir-fry (without oil) in Uncle Ben's Black Bean Sauce. Serve with cooked pasta twirls (2 oz/50 g dry weight per person).

- Spaghetti Bolognese: Use 4 oz (100 g) lean minced beef per person and dry-fry in a non-stick pan. Remove from the pan and drain away all the fat. Return the mince to the pan and add chopped onion plus Dolmio or Ragu Sauce. Serve with cooked spaghetti (2 oz/50 g dry weight per person).

- Prawn and Pasta Salad (serves 1): Mix 4 oz (100 g) cooked prawns with 4 oz (100 g) cooked pasta shells. Dress with natural yogurt mixed with tomato purée and a few drops of Tabasco sauce. Season well and sprinkle with finely chopped spring onions.

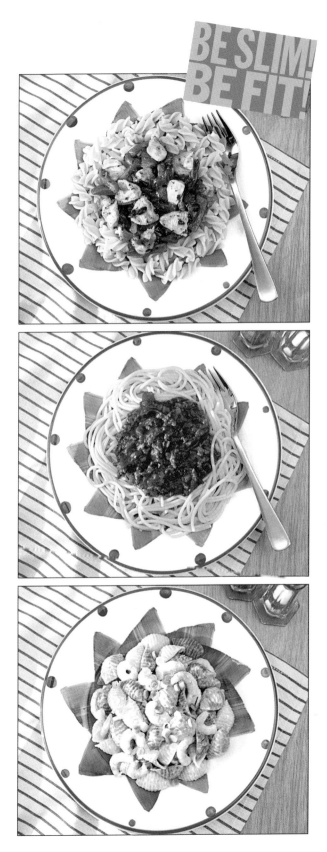

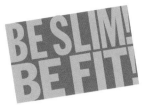

Fresh Tagliatelle with Blue Cheese Sauce

SERVES 4

As this is a vegetarian recipe, a small amount of blue cheese is acceptable.

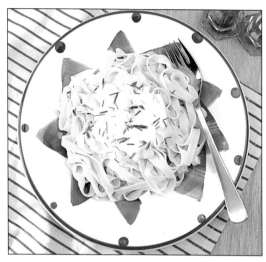

12 oz (300 g) tagliatelle
2 teaspoons arrowroot
$\frac{1}{2}$ pint (250 ml) skimmed or semi-skimmed milk
2 oz (50 g) blue cheese, crumbled
Salt and black pepper
1–2 tablespoons chopped fresh chives to garnish

Cook the tagliatelle as indicated on the packet.
Meanwhile, place the arrowroot in a small saucepan and gradually add the milk, stirring all the time. Add the blue cheese, bring the mixture to the boil and simmer for 2 minutes, making sure that the blue cheese is thoroughly melted. Season well.
Serve the sauce on a bed of the tagliatelle and sprinkle the chives on top.

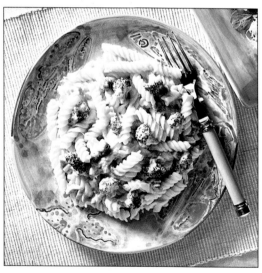

Tuna and Pasta à la King

SERVES 2

1 x 3$\frac{3}{4}$ oz (90 g) packet white sauce
8 fl oz (200 ml) skimmed or semi-skimmed milk (in addition to allowance)
4 oz (100 g) (dry weight) fusilli pasta
8 oz (200 g) can tuna in brine, drained
Salt and black pepper
4 oz (100 g) frozen broccoli, chopped

Mix the sauce powder with the milk until smooth.
Combine all the ingredients in a non-stick saucepan with 1 pint (500 ml) water and bring to the boil, stirring continuously. Once boiling, reduce the heat, cover and simmer for 10 minutes. Remove the lid and continue cooking until the mixture becomes a creamy consistency.
Serve hot with salad.

Vegetarian Dishes

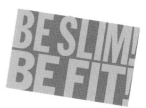

Stuffed Marrow

SERVES 4

1 medium-sized marrow
Selection of assorted vegetables, chopped
1 oz (25 g) onion, peeled and chopped
2 cloves garlic, peeled and crushed
2 tablespoons tomato purée
2 teaspoons chopped fresh rosemary
or 1 teaspoon dried rosemary
Salt and black pepper
4 oz (100 g) (dry weight) long grain rice

Skin the marrow, cut it in half lengthways and remove the seeds.

Place the vegetables, onion, garlic, tomato purée and rosemary in a saucepan with a little water. Season with salt and pepper, and cook until tender. Leave overnight for the flavour to develop.

Cook the rice in a saucepan of boiling water until tender. Mix the rice with the vegetable mixture, and spoon into the marrow halves.

Wrap the stuffed marrow in aluminium foil and bake in the oven at 200°C, 400°F, or Gas Mark 6 for one hour.

Serve with additional vegetables if desired.

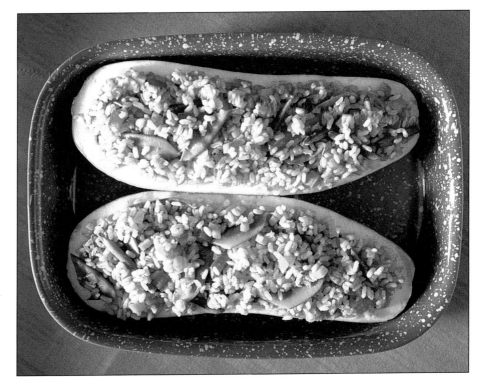

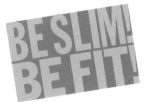

Stuffed Peppers

SERVES 1

2 peppers, red or green
1 oz (25 g) (dry weight) rice
1 teaspoon mixed herbs
1 tablespoon sweetcorn
1 tablespoon peas
1 tablespoon mushrooms, chopped
$\frac{1}{2}$ medium sized-onion,
peeled and chopped
Salt and black pepper

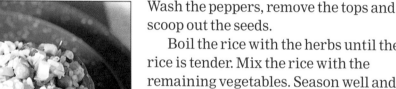

Wash the peppers, remove the tops and scoop out the seeds.

Boil the rice with the herbs until the rice is tender. Mix the rice with the remaining vegetables. Season well and pile the mixture into the peppers. Place on a baking tray and bake in a preheated oven at 160°C, 325°F, or Gas Mark 3 for 20 minutes.

Serve with additional vegetables if desired.

Sweetcorn and Potato Fritters

SERVES 2

8 oz (200 g) sweetcorn, cooked
8 oz (200 g) potatoes, cooked
1 egg white
2 tablespoons chopped, fresh parsley
1 teaspoon mustard

Mash the potatoes and mix with the sweetcorn.

Whisk the egg white and stir into the mixture, then add the parsley and the mustard. Wet your hands and form the mixture into small cakes (approximately $2\frac{3}{4}$ in/7 cm in diameter).

Dry-fry the cakes in a non-stick frying pan until golden brown on each side.

Serve with additional vegetables if desired.

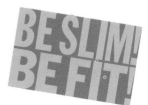

Vegetable Kebabs

SERVES 2

1 green pepper, deseeded and chopped into
$^3/_4$ in (2 cm) squares
1 red pepper, deseeded and chopped into
$^3/_4$ in (2 cm) squares
1 large Spanish onion, peeled and
cut into large pieces or
6 oz (150 g) small button onions, peeled
8 oz (200 g) button mushrooms, washed
4 courgettes, coarsely sliced
1 lb (400 g) average-sized fresh tomatoes,
cut in half
1 teaspoon thyme
Cayenne pepper

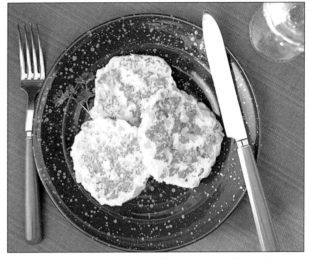

Sweetcorn and Potato Fritters

Vegetable Kebabs with sweetcorn and rice

Thread the vegetable pieces
alternately on to 4 skewers to
make 4 kebabs.

Cover a baking sheet with
aluminium foil and place the
kebabs on to the foil. Sprinkle
with thyme. Wrap the foil
around the kebabs to make a
parcel and cook in a
preheated oven at 180°C,
350°F, or Gas Mark 4 for 35
minutes.

Remove from the oven.
Unwrap the foil and place
the kebabs on a bed of hot
sweetcorn (4 oz/100 g)
mixed with boiled rice
(4 oz/50 g dry weight).

Return to the oven
for one minute. Serve
hot.

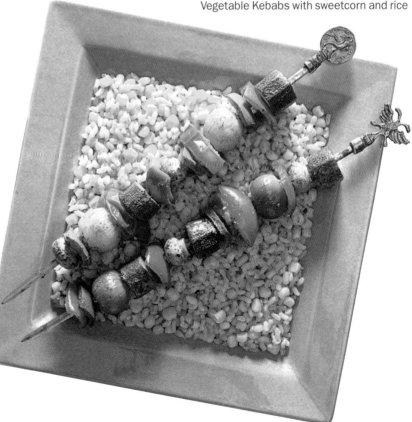

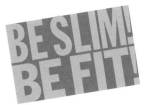

Vegetarian Spaghetti Bolognese

SERVES 4

3 oz (75 g) (dry weight) soya mince
3 oz (75 g) mushrooms
15 oz (375 g) canned tomatoes
1 teaspoon vegetable or yeast extract
$\frac{1}{2}$ green pepper, deseeded and finely chopped
1 teaspoon oregano
2 cloves garlic, peeled and crushed
1 tablespoon gravy powder
6 oz (150 g) egg-free spaghetti
Chopped fresh herbs to garnish

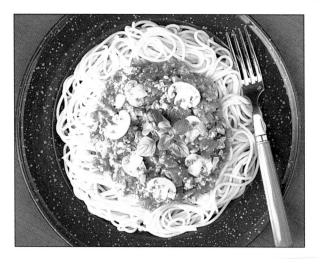

Presoak the soya mince in two cups of boiling water and leave to stand for 10 minutes. Drain.

Place the soya mince, mushrooms, tomatoes, pepper, vegetable or yeast extract, oregano and garlic in a saucepan with a little water. Cover, and simmer for 10 minutes.

Mix the gravy powder with a little cold water and stir into the sauce mixture.

Boil the spaghetti for 10–20 minutes until tender. Drain and place in a serving dish. Pour the sauce on top and garnish with fresh herbs if desired.

Mixed Bean Hotpot

SERVES 4

Selection of canned beans (1 lb / 400 g total weight)
e.g. red or white kidney beans, borlotti beans, butter beans,
pinto beans, blackeye beans, flageolet beans
4 oz (100 g) green beans
1 x 16 oz (400 g) can tomatoes
1 clove garlic, peeled and crushed
1 teaspoon mixed herbs
Salt and black pepper to taste
1 lb (400 g) potatoes, par-boiled
4 oz (100 g) half-fat Cheddar-type cheese, grated

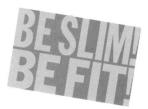

Drain and rinse the canned beans and place together with the green beans in an ovenproof casserole dish.

Mix together the tomatoes, garlic, herbs and seasonings. Pour over the beans and mix well.

Thinly slice the par-boiled potatoes and lay the slices on top of the bean mixture. Sprinkle with the grated cheese.

Bake in a preheated oven at 160°C, 325°F, or Gas Mark 3 for one hour until the potatoes are cooked.

Serve with additional vegetables or salad.

Tofu Burgers

SERVES 2

16 oz (400 g) medium tofu
2 oz (50 g) oats
$^1/_2$ teaspoon ground cumin
1 teaspoon chilli powder
1 clove garlic, peeled and crushed
1 onion, peeled and very finely chopped
Salt and black pepper to taste

Preheat a non-stick frying pan.

Place the tofu in a large bowl and mash well with a fork. Add the remaining ingredients and mix well.

Shape the mixture into 6 burgers and place in the frying pan. Cook until the burgers are brown on both sides, turning them carefully.

Serve in burger buns (2 oz/50 g bun per person) with unlimited salad.

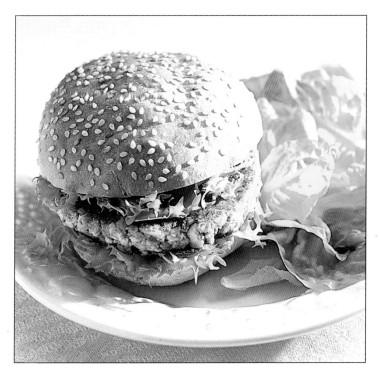

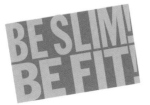

Spicy Chickpea Casserole

SERVES 4

8 oz (200 g) (dry weight) chickpeas, soaked overnight
1 medium onion, peeled and chopped
1 x 16 oz (400 g) can tomatoes
$^1/_2$ teaspoon coriander
2 heaped teaspoons cumin seeds or 1 teaspoon ground cumin
$^1/_2$ teaspoon chilli powder
Salt and black pepper to taste
8 oz (200 g) mushrooms, sliced

Fast-boil the chickpeas for 10 minutes and then simmer for a further 20–25 minutes until fairly soft.

Meanwhile place the onion and tomatoes into a medium saucepan. Add the coriander, cumin, chilli and seasoning. Bring to the boil and simmer gently for 10 minutes.

When the chickpeas are almost cooked, drain and rinse with boiling water, then stir into the tomato mixture. Add the mushrooms and simmer for a further 5 minutes.

Serve with boiled brown rice (2 oz/50 g dry weight per person) and unlimited vegetables.

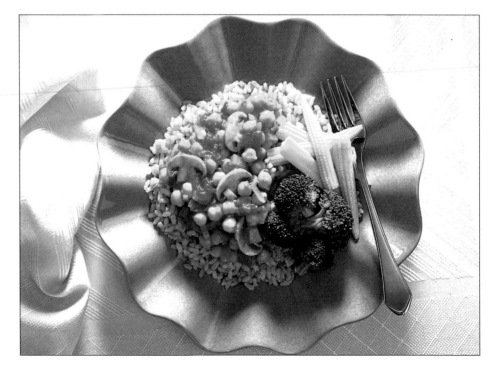

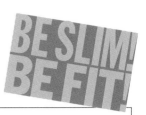

Quick and Easy Vegetarian Dishes

- Batchelor's Beanfeast Bolognese-style Soya in Rich Tomato Sauce served with 2 oz (50 g) (dry weight) cooked spaghetti.
- Batchelor's Beanfeast Soya Mince with Onion in a Savoury Gravy served with unlimited potatoes and vegetables.
- Batchelor's Beanfeast Mexican Chilli served with 2 oz (50 g) (dry weight) boiled brown rice, plus mixed salad.
- Asda World Bistro Vegetable Chilli (392 g can serves 2) served with boiled brown rice (2 oz/50 g dry weight per person), plus salad.
- Vegetable Chop Suey: Dry-fry in a little soy sauce chopped carrots, snow peas, chopped water chestnuts, bamboo shoots and beansprouts. When barely cooked, serve with 2 oz (50 g) (dry weight) boiled brown rice and extra soy sauce.
- Vegetable Chilli: Mix 8 oz (200 g) peas with 8 oz (200 g) baked beans and cook in contents of 1 small jar any cook-in chilli sauce. Serve with 2 oz (50 g) (dry weight) boiled brown rice.

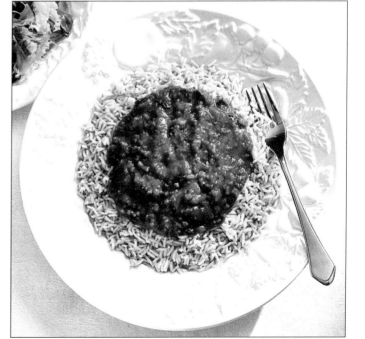

Batchelor's Beanfeast Soya Mince with Onion in a Savoury Gravy

Batchelor's Beanfeast Mexican Chilli

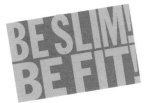

Vegetable Bake

SERVES 1

Selection of vegetables (e.g. carrots, parsnips,
beans, cabbage, leeks, onions)
3 tablespoons stuffing mix
1 teaspoon mixed herbs
6 oz (150 g) potatoes, cooked
$\frac{1}{4}$ pint (125 ml) vegetable stock
Salt and black pepper to taste

Slice the vegetables and place in layers in a small dish. Sprinkle with the
stuffing mix and mixed herbs. Slice the cooked potatoes and lay the
slices across the top of the dish. Pour the vegetable stock over and
season well.

Cook in a preheated oven at 200°C, 400°F, or Gas Mark 6 until golden
brown on top.

Chickpea and Fennel Casserole

SERVES 2

1 clove garlic
6 oz (150 g) celery
6 oz (150 g) whole green beans
2 teaspoons fennel seeds
3 oz (75 g) cooked chickpeas
1 oz (25 g) bulgar wheat
$\frac{1}{2}$ pint (250 ml) vegetable stock
2 tablespoons soy sauce
Salt and freshly ground black pepper
2 tablespoons chopped fresh mint to garnish

Crush the garlic, dice the celery and chop the green beans. Crush the
fennel seeds.

Cook the chickpeas, bulgar wheat, celery, fennel and garlic gently in
a little stock for about 5 minutes. Add the remaining ingredients,
excluding the mint, and simmer for 20 minutes.

Garnish with the fresh mint and serve with unlimited vegetables.

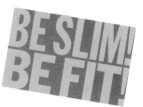

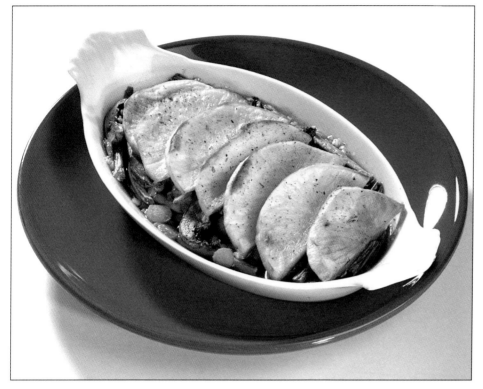

Vegetable Bake

Chickpea and Fennel
Casserole

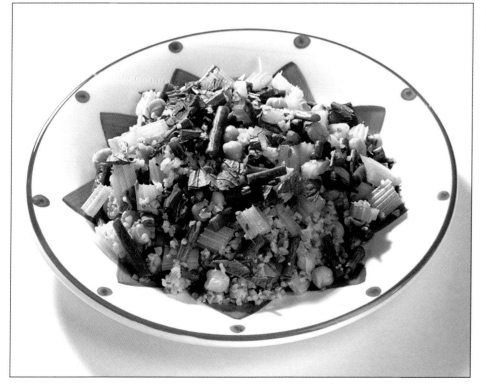

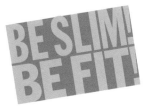

Quick and Easy Desserts

- 5 oz (125 g) jelly with 1 small chopped banana, plus 1 oz (25 g) Wall's 'Too Good To Be True' ice cream.
- 6 oz (150 g) fresh fruit salad topped with 1 tablespoon yogurt.
- 1 pear, peeled and poached in a little red wine and artificial sweetener, served with 1 teaspoon fromage frais.
- 2 brown Ryvitas spread with Marmite and topped with cottage cheese.

Banana and Kiwi Salad

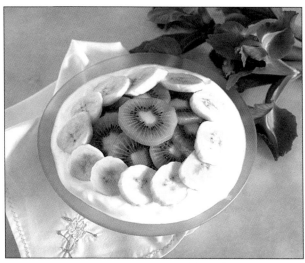

- Banana and Kiwi Salad: 1 large banana and 2 kiwi fruits, peeled and sliced, plus 5 oz (125 g) fromage frais.
- 1 Shape Twinpot yogurt.
- 4 oz (100 g) 'Too Good To Be True' ice cream.
- 1 banana and 1 pear.
- 8 oz (200 g) cherries.
- 8 oz (200 g) fresh raspberries topped with 2½ oz (62.5 g) diet yogurt.
- 4 dried apricots, soaked in black or fruit tea overnight. Add a pinch of cinnamon and serve with 5 oz (125 g) diet yogurt.
- 4 oz (100 g) sorbet (any flavour).
- 5 oz (125 g) fromage frais with 2 oz (50 g) any fruit.
- Heat 4 oz (100 g) canned cherries and serve with 2 oz (50 g) 'Too Good To Be True' ice cream.
- 1 Shape yogurt plus 1 banana.
- 2 oz (50 g) 'Too Good To Be True' ice cream plus 1 oz (25 g) Jordan's Crunch cereal sprinkled on top.
- 2 oz (50 g) 'Too Good To Be True' ice cream sprinkled with ½ oz (12.5 g) bran flakes or Fruit and Fibre cereal.
- Meringue biscuit plus 2 oz (50 g) fresh fruit salad and 2 oz (50 g) fromage frais.

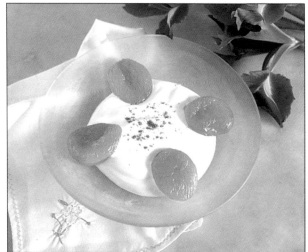

Dried apricots with diet yogurt

- Meringue basket topped with 2 oz (50 g) 'Too Good To Be True' double toffee ice cream.
- 4 oz (100 g) strawberries plus 4 oz (100 g) raspberries topped with 2 teaspoons fromage frais.

- 4 oz (100 g) cottage cheese mixed with 1 tablespoon strawberry jam.
- $\frac{1}{2}$ orange, peeled and sliced, plus $\frac{1}{2}$ banana, peeled and sliced, and 6 grapes, served with 2 oz (50 g) cottage cheese.
- 5 oz (125 g) natural yogurt mixed with $\frac{1}{2}$ oz (12.5 g) muesli.
- Melon and Strawberries: Deseed $\frac{1}{2}$ ogen melon and fill the centre with strawberries.
- Melon Salad: Mix together cubes of honeydew, ogen and water melon and top with fromage frais.
- Oranges in Cointreau: Peel and slice 4 oranges and leave to soak in 4 tablespoons Cointreau liqueur.
- $\frac{1}{4}$ pint (125 ml) jelly plus $\frac{1}{2}$ banana, sliced, and $2\frac{1}{2}$ oz (62.5 g) diet yogurt.

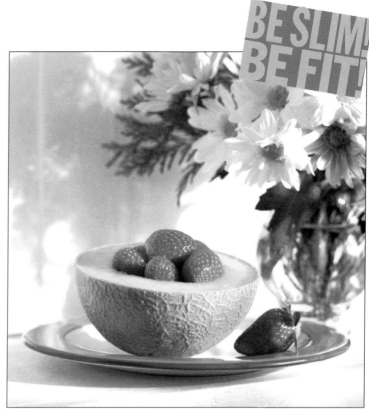

Melon and Strawberries

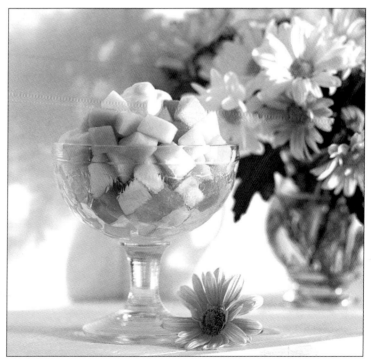

Melon Salad

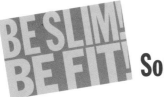

Sorbet Specials

Pineapple and Orange Sorbet

SERVES 6

Small can pineapple in natural juice
1 orange, peeled and chopped
8 fl oz (200 ml) fresh orange juice
Liquid artificial sweetener to taste
2 egg whites

Crush the pineapple well and mix with the chopped orange and orange juice. Sweeten to taste. Place in a plastic container in the freezer and freeze until half-frozen.

Whisk the egg whites until stiff. Turn out the half-frozen mixture into a bowl and fold in the whisked egg whites.

Return the mixture to the freezer until firm.

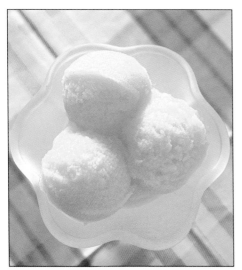

Pineapple and Orange Sorbet

Kiwi Fruit Sorbet

SERVES 4

5 kiwi fruits, peeled and thickly sliced
2 tablespoons Cointreau
4 oz (100 g) caster sugar
1 egg white
Fresh fruit to decorate

Place the kiwi fruits in a blender with the Cointreau. Pour the mixture into a bowl and freeze for about 2 hours.

Tip the mixture into a fresh bowl and whisk to break up the crystals. Beat the egg white until stiff and fold into the fruit purée. Place in a decorative bowl and freeze.

Remove from the freezer half an hour before serving. Decorate with fresh fruit of your choice.

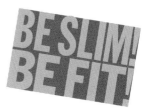

Apple and Lime Sorbet

SERVES 4–6

3 cooking apples, peeled, cored and grated
2 tablespoons lime juice
4 tablespoons concentrated apple juice
4 teaspoons honey
2 egg whites

Mix together the apples, lime juice, apple juice and honey and make up to $^3/_4$ pint (275 ml) with cold water. Freeze until slushy.

Whisk the egg whites until stiff then stir into the apple mixture and return to the freezer.

Remove from the freezer 25 minutes before serving.

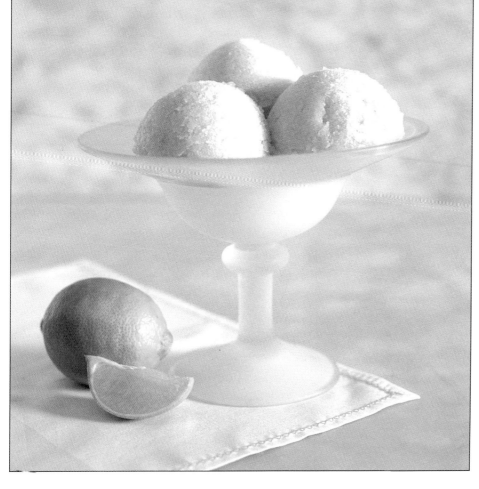

Apple and Lime Sorbet

Fruity Desserts

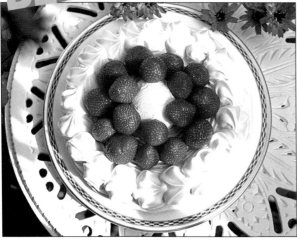

- Meringue with Strawberries and Ice Cream: Use bought meringue baskets or make your own (see recipe for Pears in Meringue) and top with 4 oz (100 g) strawberries and 2 oz (50 g) Wall's 'Too Good To Be True' ice cream.

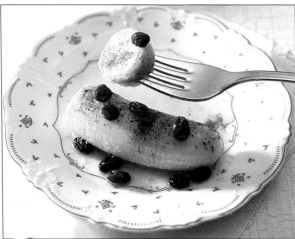

- Baked Banana: Peel and slice 1 banana and place in a shallow dish. Sprinkle 1 teaspoon brown sugar, 10 raisins and a pinch cinnamon over. Add 4 tablespoons water (and 1 tablespoon rum if desired) and bake at 180°C, 350°F, or Gas Mark 4 for 30 minutes.

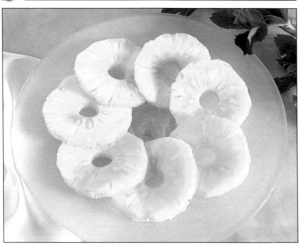

- Pineapple in Kirsch: Sprinkle 1 sherry glass Kirsch over pineapple rings and leave to marinate in the refrigerator for 12 hours. Turn the fruit regularly to ensure even flavouring.

Baked Stuffed Apple

SERVES 1

1 oz (25 g) dried fruit
1 teaspoon honey
1 large apple, cored
2 tablespoons natural yogurt
or fromage frais

Mix together the dried fruit and honey and pile into the centre of the apple. Bake in a moderate oven (200°C, 400°F, or Gas Mark 6) for about 30 minutes.

Serve with the yogurt or fromage frais.

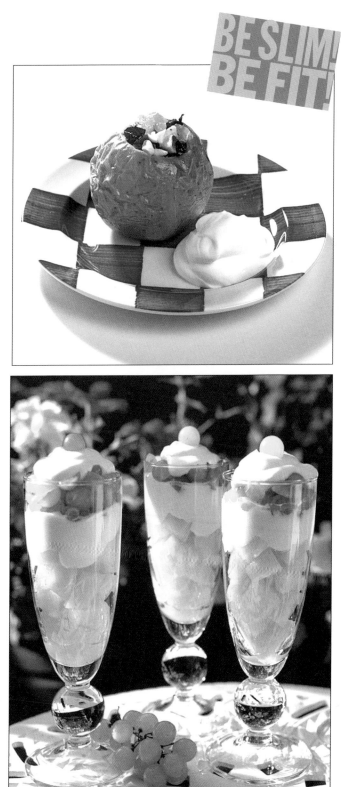

Melon Sundae

SERVES 4

16 oz (400 g) melon flesh
10 oz (250 g) diet yogurt
8 oz (200 g) green grapes

Finely chop the melon flesh and place in tall glasses. Spoon sufficient yogurt over to cover the melon.

Wash the grapes and reserve 4 for decoration. Halve and seed the remainder and divide them equally between the glasses, placing the grapes on top of the yogurt. Top with the remainder of the yogurt and keep chilled until ready to serve.

To decorate, place a grape on top of each glass.

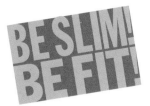

Oranges Grand Marnier with Yogurt Sauce

SERVES 4

1 wine glass white wine or orange juice
1 sherry glass Grand Marnier liqueur
1 tablespoon demerara sugar
or liquid artificial sweetener if preferred
6 oranges

For the sauce
2 tablespoons Grand Marnier
8 oz (200 g) natural yogurt

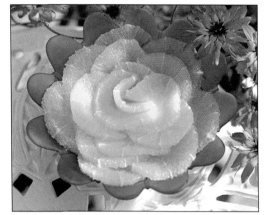

Heat the white wine or orange juice with the liqueur
in a saucepan. Add the sugar, bring to the boil and
simmer until the sugar has dissolved. Leave to cool.
　Peel and slice the oranges and place in the cool
liquid. Chill in a refrigerator for at least 12 hours.
　Just before serving, mix the yogurt with the 2
tablespoons Grand Marnier and serve separately as

Tropical Fruit Salad

SERVES 4

6 oz (150 g) fresh pineapple
1 mango
1 banana
1 kiwi fruit
2 oranges
4 oz (100 g) seedless grapes
6 fl oz (150 ml) tropical fruit juice
2 fl oz (50 ml) fruit liqueur
(e.g. Grand Marnier, Cointreau or Kirsch)

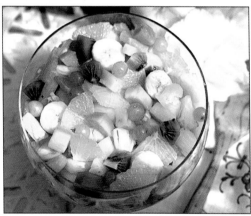

Skin and cube the pineapple. Peel and slice the mango, banana and kiwi
fruit into bite-sized pieces. Peel the oranges and remove all the pith,
then chop into small pieces.
　Mix all the ingredients together in a bowl and place in the
refrigerator. Serve within one hour to avoid discolouration.

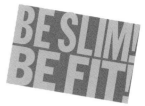

Pears in Meringue

SERVES 6

6 ripe dessert pears, peeled but left whole
$\frac{1}{2}$ pint (250 ml) apple juice

For the meringue
3 egg whites
6 oz (150 g) caster sugar

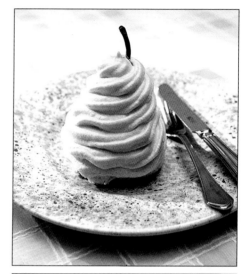

Place the pears and apple juice in a saucepan and cook until just tender. Remove the pears from the pan and cut a slice off the bottom of each to enable them to sit in a dish without falling over. Place them, well spaced out, in an ovenproof dish.

To make the meringue, whisk the egg whites until they are firm and stand in peaks, then whisk in 1 tablespoon of the caster sugar for one minute. Fold in the remainder of the sugar with a metal spoon, cutting the egg whites rather than mixing them.

Place the egg white and sugar mixture into a large piping bag with a metal nozzle (any pattern) and pipe a pyramid around each pear, starting from the base and working upwards. Place in a preheated oven and bake at 160°C, 325°F, or Gas Mark 3 until firm and golden.

Serve hot or cold.

Fruit Sundae

SERVES 2

8 oz (200 g) fruit (blackberries, raspberries, strawberries or a mixture)
6 drops liquid artificial sweetener
5 oz (125 g) natural yogurt
1 egg white
Angelica and vermouth (optional)

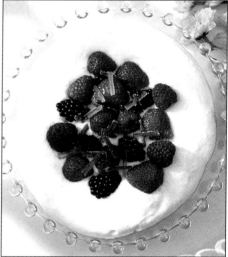

Stir the fruit, sweetener and yogurt together thoroughly.

Whisk the egg white until stiff and fold into the fruit mixture. Spoon into serving glasses. Top with angelica and vermouth if desired.

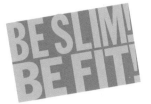

Apple and Blackcurrant Whip

SERVES 4

1 lb cooking apples
2 fl oz (50 ml) water
Saccharin or liquid artificial sweetener to taste
2 egg whites
2 tablespoons low-calorie blackcurrant jam
or 4 oz (100 g) fresh or frozen blackcurrants

Peel, core and slice the apples and cook in the water until they become a thick pulp. Add the saccharin or sweetener and set aside to cool.

Whisk the egg whites until stiff and fold gently into the cooled apple purée. Pile into individual sundae dishes or a medium-sized serving dish.

Swirl the blackcurrant jam or fruit on top to give a ripple effect.

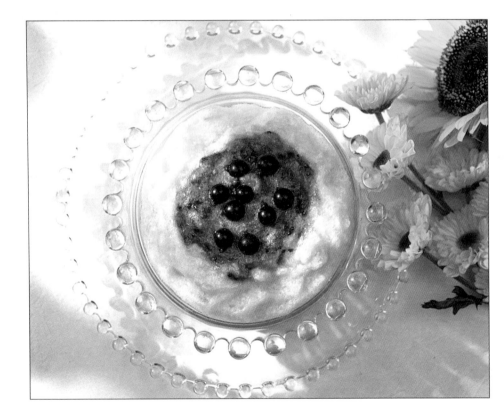

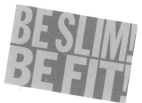

Raspberry Mousse

SERVES 4

8 oz (200 g) fresh or frozen raspberries
or 7 oz (175 g) canned raspberries in natural juice
4 oz (100 g) natural apple juice
Liquid artificial sweetener
(approximately 15 drops)
1 teaspoon gelatine
2 egg whites
4 teaspoons raspberry yogurt
12 fresh raspberries to decorate

Place the raspberries and apple juice in a liquidiser and blend until smooth. Add liquid sweetener to taste.

Dissolve the gelatine in 3 teaspoons of water in a cup over very hot water. Add to the raspberry purée and stir well.

Whisk the egg whites until they form peaks. Fold into the purée.

Pour the mixture into 4 tall sundae glasses. Decorate each with a teaspoon of raspberry yogurt and 3 fresh raspberries just before serving.

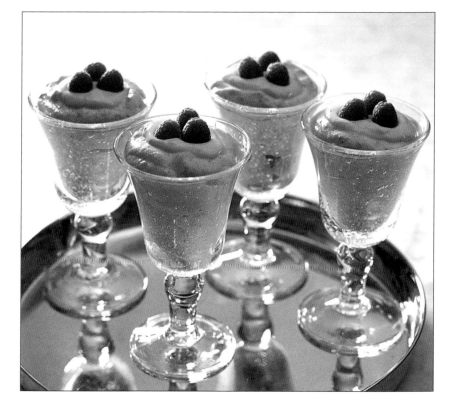

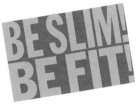

Family Favourites

Low-fat Pancakes

SERVES 4

This recipe makes 8 pancakes, allowing 2 pancakes per person.

4 oz (100 g) plain flour
Pinch salt
1 egg yolk
$\frac{1}{2}$ pint (250 ml) skimmed or semi-skimmed milk
(in addition to allowance)
$\frac{1}{2}$ teaspoon melted butter or oil

Sift the flour together with the salt in a bowl and make a well in the centre. Pour the egg yolk into the well and stir into the flour very carefully, adding half the milk slowly and stirring all the time. Stir in the melted butter or oil and beat until smooth. Add the remaining milk and leave the mixture to stand for 20–30 minutes. The batter should be the consistency of thick cream. If it is too thick, add extra milk.

Preheat a non-stick frying pan with the butter or oil and take 1 tablespoon of batter for each pancake. Tilt the pan as you pour in the batter so that the batter spreads evenly across the bottom of the pan. Cook until the underneath of the pancake is a golden brown colour, then wedge a wooden spatula around the edge of the pancake to raise it slightly. Flip the pancake over and cook for about 15 seconds on the other side.

Serve immediately with fresh orange or lemon juice and honey or brown sugar.

Low-fat Trifle

SERVES 4

1 packet sugar-free jelly
2 medium-sized bananas, peeled and sliced
17 oz (425 g) carton low-fat custard
10 oz (250 g) vanilla virtually fat-free yogurt

Make up the jelly as instructed on the packet in a large dish. Add the bananas and leave to set.

Once set, cover the jelly with the low-fat custard, then smooth the yogurt over the top.

THE BE SLIM! BE FIT! EATING PLAN

Swiss Roll Meringue

SERVES 6–8

4 egg whites
6 oz (150 g) caster sugar
1 teaspoon each icing sugar and caster
sugar for sprinkling

For the filling
12 oz (300 g) raspberries, puréed
½ pint (250 ml) fromage frais
2 teaspoons gelatine dissolved in
2 tablespoons hot water

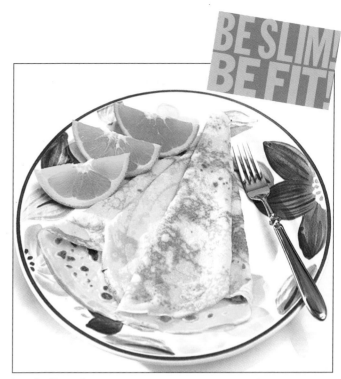
Low-fat Pancakes

Whisk the egg whites until stiff. Whisk in 3 oz (75 g) of the caster sugar and add the vanilla essence.

Line a large Swiss roll tin with baking parchment. Spread the meringue mixture evenly into the tin.

Bake in a preheated oven at 160°C, 325°F, or Gas Mark 3 for 12 minutes. Reduce the oven temperature to 150°C, 300°F, or Gas Mark 2 and bake for a further 15 minutes.

Tip the meringue carefully on to a separate sheet of baking parchment. Sprinkle liberally with the icing sugar and caster sugar, and leave to cool.

To make the filling, freeze two-thirds of the raspberry purée until it forms crystals. Beat the fromage frais and gelatine together. Leave to chill until the mixture starts to thicken and set.

Add the semi-frozen raspberry purée to the fromage frais and then spread the mixture over the meringue. Roll up like a Swiss roll and freeze.

Serve with the remaining raspberry purée.

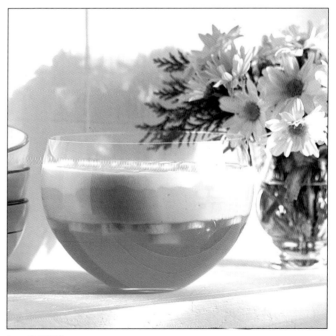
Low-fat Trifle

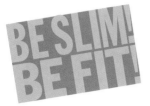

Diet Rice Pudding

SERVES 4

1 pint (500 ml) skimmed milk (in addition to allowance)
1 oz (25 g) pudding rice
Artificial sweetener to taste (approximately 15 saccharin
tablets or 20 drops liquid sweetener)
Pinch nutmeg (optional)

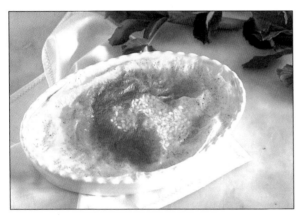

Place all the ingredients except the nutmeg in an ovenproof dish. Sprinkle the nutmeg over the top, if desired. Bake in a preheated oven for 2–2½ hours at 150°C, 300°F, or Gas Mark 2.

If the pudding is still sloppy 30–40 minutes before it is to be eaten, raise the oven temperature to 160°C, 325°F, or Gas Mark 3.

Serve hot or cold. If you intend to serve cold, remove from the oven while still very moist as it will become stiffer and drier when cool.

Banana and Sultana Cake

1 SERVING = ½ IN / 1.25 CM SLICE

This is an economical recipe because very ripe bananas can often be purchased cheaply. Because of the number of portions that can be served from this loaf, the egg content need not be included in your allowance of 2 eggs per week.

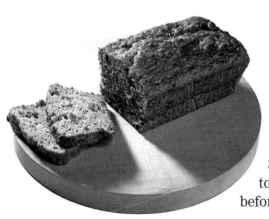

1 lb 3 oz (475 g) ripe bananas (approx. 5 large), peeled
2 beaten eggs
6 oz (150 g) brown sugar
4 oz (100 g) sultanas
8 oz (200 g) self-raising flour

Mash the bananas and add the eggs, sugar and sultanas. Mix well, then stir in the flour. Place in a lined 2 lb (800 g) loaf tin or cake tin. Bake for one hour and 15 minutes in a preheated oven at 180°C, 350°F, or Gas Mark 4. Remove from the oven and leave to cool. When cool, store in an air-tight tin for 24 hours before serving.

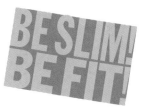

Apple and Blackberry Cake

MAKES 10–12 SLICES

1 cup All Bran cereal
$^1/_2$ cup skimmed or semi-skimmed milk
(in addition to allowance)
1 cup sugar
1 cup self-raising flour
1 cup grated Bramley apple
3 oz (75 g) blackberries

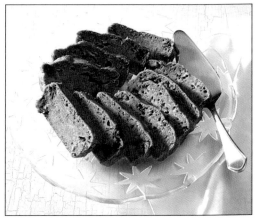

Soak the All Bran in the milk for about 2 hours until soft. Add the sugar, flour and grated apple, mixing well. Fold in the blackberries and pour into a lined 2 lb (800 g) loaf tin.

Bake in the centre of the oven at 150°C, 300°F, or Gas Mark 2 for 2 hours.

Leave to cool. When cold, cut into slices.

Prune Cake

SERVES 8–10

You will find that this cake has a slightly chewy texture to it.

6 oz (150 g) self-raising flour
6 oz (150 g) caster sugar
3 beaten eggs
1 heaped teaspoon mixed spice (cinnamon or ginger)
4 oz (100 g) stoned prunes, soaked in black tea
overnight and drained
Icing sugar (optional)

Place all the ingredients in a food processor and blend well.

Pour the mixture into a lined and lightly greased rectangular cake tin.

Bake in a preheated oven at 200°C, 400°F, or Gas Mark 6 for approximately 30–35 minutes. Remove from the oven and leave to cool in the tin.

While the cake is still warm pour a weak solution of icing sugar mixed with water over the top if desired.

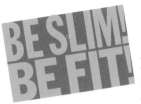

The Be Slim! Be Fit! Exercise Plan

My Be Slim! Be Fit! Workout is specially designed to help you burn fat, tone up and improve your fitness, flexibility and energy level.

The workout consists of four sections: warm-up, aerobic, toning and the cool-down and stretch.

The warm-up starts with some mobilising movements to loosen the joints, warm the muscles and prepare the body for exercise by rehearsing the movements that are to follow. These are followed by some preparatory stretches which encourage the blood flow to the muscles and makes them more pliable. Preparing the heart and lungs for the additional work they will be undertaking, and stretching out the muscles we will be working helps enhance our performance as well as prevent injury and soreness.

The aerobic section consists of a moderate level workout which strengthens the heart and lungs by increasing the demand for oxygen in the body in order to sustain the activity. It also helps us burn fat as the body calls upon its reserves of fat for the additional energy required. Remember, for aerobic exercise to be effective, you need to work out at a level that causes you to be mildly breathless and perspiring but still able to carry on a conversation.

The toning section is divided into exercises for the upper body (chest, arms, upper back), the middle body (tummy, waist, back) and the lower body (bottom, legs and thighs). For all-round toning benefits you can practise all of these exercises, or you can choose to focus on a specific area of the body.

For maximum effect each toning exercise should be performed slowly and rhythmically and repeated to the point where you feel mild discomfort, but not pain, to allow the muscle to become slightly fatigued. This enables the muscle to tighten and become stronger. As muscle requires calories to sustain it, the more muscle mass we have, the more calories we will burn.

Although guidelines are given, the number of repetitions you are able to do will be determined by your individual ability. Always work at your own pace and just do as many as you are able, then rest for a few

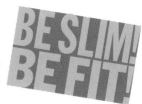

moments and repeat the exercise. As the days go by, you'll find you are able to increase the number of repetitions in order to challenge your body further.

After 'working' the muscles we need to stretch them to help them relax and return to their normal state. The cool-down stretches will also help prevent injury or soreness as well as improve your flexibility and range of movement. Even on those days when you don't do the full work-out it's a good idea to work on improving your flexibility by practising these stretches.

Practise the Be Slim! Be Fit! Workout as often as possible, but always allow one day a week to rest. Try to set aside a certain period of time each day for your exercise session so that it becomes a habit. Always start with the warm-up and finish with the cool-down stretches to get the best from your workout. It will have a beneficial effect on your health, your body and your physical shape, so please do not rush your workout.

The exercises should be performed on a well-cushioned carpet, or alternatively use a rug or foam mat to protect you from a hard floor. If possible, exercise to your favourite music. The beat of the music will give you a momentum and you'll find the whole experience much more enjoyable, which will encourage you to continue for longer.

On those days when you find your schedule is particularly hectic you can choose to do the Five-minute Workout (see pages 130 to 135) or simply practise the cool-down stretches to work on improving your flexibility. The Five-minute Workout consists of a warm-up followed by a short tone and stretch routine. You will need to combine this with some aerobic activity such as brisk walking or swimming for overall fitness and fat-burning benefits.

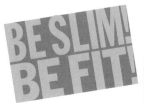

Ten Tips For Exercising

1 If you have any doubts about your health, always check with your doctor before you start exercising.

2 Always wear the appropriate clothing such as leggings and a T shirt. Cushioned training shoes are essential for aerobic exercise.

3 Set aside a particular time each day for your workout so that you get into a routine and it becomes a habit. Don't expect instant results, but you'll be surprised how quickly you'll see a difference.

4 Always start out gently and build up gradually. You will enjoy greater benefits in the long term if you don't attempt too much too soon. If you do, you'll ache so much you'll give up.

5 Always warm up before exercising and cool down afterwards.

6 Never exercise on a full stomach. However, eating some carbohydrate before you undertake aerobic exercise will encourage maximum fat burning. If you go to a class straight from work and you ate last at lunchtime, eat a banana half an hour before you work out. It will enhance your energy output considerably.

7 Never overwork or overstretch your body. Look for warning signals such as feeling faint, nausea and so on. Stop immediately if you feel any pain and, if necessary, consult a doctor.

8 When undertaking aerobic exercise, remember that for maximum fat burning you should only be sweating mildly and a little out of breath – not fit to drop!

9 Toning exercises increase muscle mass, which in turn increases your metabolic rate. All movements should be slow and controlled, never jerky or hurried, and you should actually feel the muscles working.

10 Working out to your favourite music can provide added motivation and enjoyment. If you don't enjoy exercising alone, go along to a class to work out with others and enjoy the camaraderie (see page 160).

The Be Slim! Be Fit! Workout

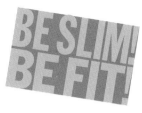

Warm-up

Shoulder Rolls

Stand with feet shoulder-width apart, knees slightly bent, tummy tight and shoulders back. Roll one shoulder backwards in a large circle. Do 8, then repeat on the other side.

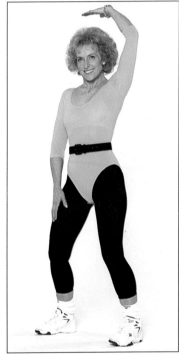

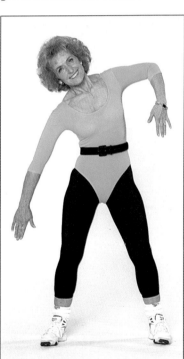

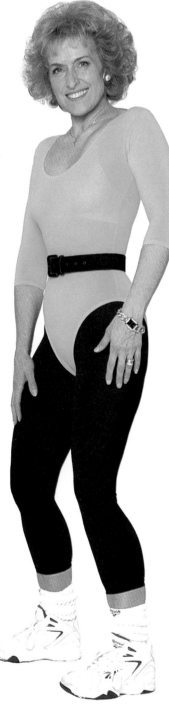

Extended Shoulder Rolls

Rotate alternate arms backwards as if brushing your hair, transferring your weight from one foot to the other. Do 16.

Side Bends

With feet a comfortable distance apart, lean to one side, keeping the hips fixed and knees slightly bent. Repeat to the other side. Do 8 to each side.

Knee Lifts

Standing tall, lift alternate knees to below waist level. Do 16.

Hip Rolls

Stand with feet hip-distance apart with knees slightly bent. Now roll the hips round in a full circle, keeping your tummy tight. Do 8 in one direction, then change direction and repeat.

Knee Bends

Stand with feet shoulder-width apart. Now imagine you are going to sit in a chair by bending from the knees and hips. Keep your back straight and your knees in line with the toes. Come up again and repeat. Do 12.

Ankle/Elbow Mobiliser

Tap the heel and then the toe of one foot, alternately flexing and straightening your elbows. Stand tall throughout and keep the knee of the supporting leg slightly bent. Do 8, then repeat on the other leg.

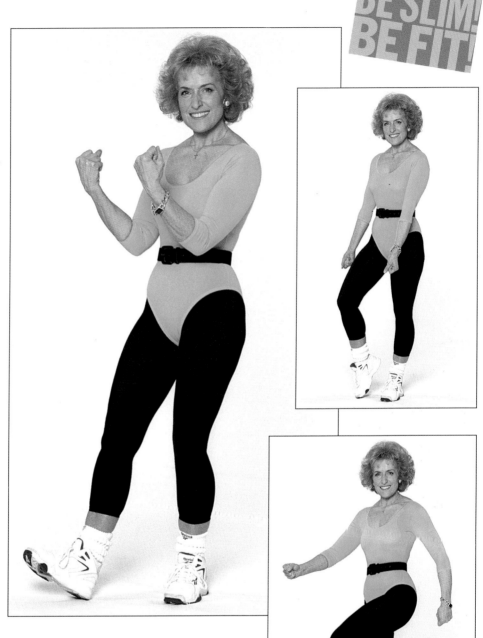

Marching

March briskly on the spot. Let the arms swing naturally and ensure the whole foot makes contact with the floor. Keep your head up and tummy tight. Sustain for 2 minutes.

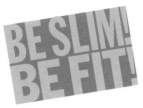

Warm-up Stretches

Chest Stretch

Take your arms behind you and clasp the hands. Now squeeze your shoulder blades close together. Keep the elbows slightly bent. Hold for 8 seconds then release.

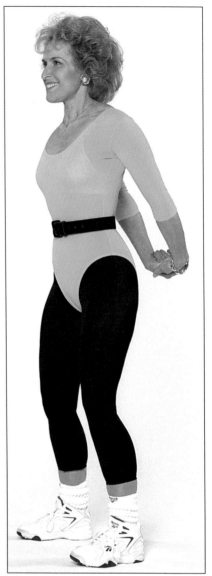

Upper Back Stretch

Bring your hands together in front of your chest. Lower your head and press your upper back away from your hands. Hold for 8 seconds then release.

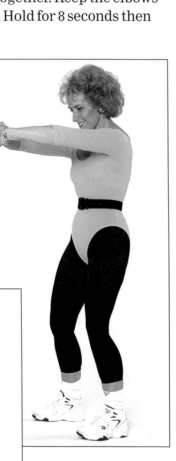

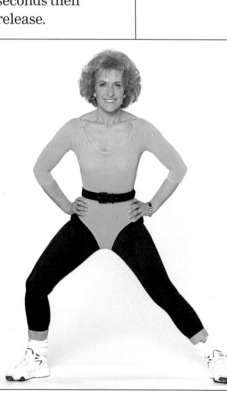

Inner Thigh Stretch

Take the legs wide apart. Bend one knee in line with the toes. Turn the foot of the straight leg forwards. Keep looking ahead and try not to lean forwards. Hold for 8 seconds, then change legs and repeat on the other side.

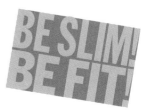

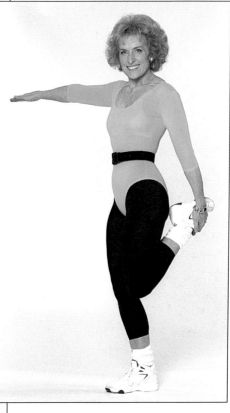

Back of Thigh Stretch

Bend one knee and place the other leg slightly in front. Keeping the front leg straight with hands placed in the middle of the thighs, lean forwards. Hold for 8 seconds, then change legs and repeat.

Front of Thigh Stretch

Take your weight on to one leg (hold on to a chair for support if necessary) and lift the other leg in front to take hold of the ankle. Now draw the knees in line with each other and push the hips slightly forwards. Hold for 8 seconds, then change legs and repeat.

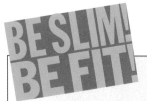

Calf Stretch

Shift your weight on to your front leg and bend the knee. Keep the back leg straight with toes pointing forwards and heel of the back foot firmly down. Hold for 8 seconds, then change legs and repeat.

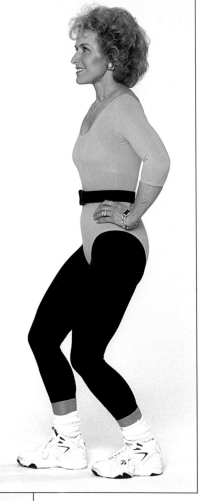

Lower Calf Stretch

Bring the back foot closer to the front foot and, keeping both legs bent, take your weight on to the back leg, tucking the seat under. Hold for 8 seconds, then change legs and repeat.

Aerobic

Marching

March on the spot, swinging your arms naturally. Stand tall throughout and ensure the whole foot makes contact with the floor. Do 32.

Circling Squats

Take the feet wide apart. Bending from the knees, cross your arms down in front of you. Continue to make a large circle with the arms as you straighten the legs and bring your arms above the head. Try to keep your back lifted and your head up at all times. Take care not to lock out the knees as you straighten the legs. Do 12.

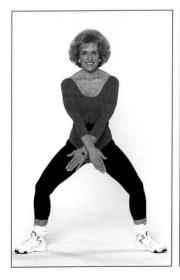

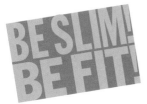

Ski Swings

Stand with feet hip-distance apart. Start with your arms in front and slightly raised. Now swing the arms down by your sides and slightly to the back of you, at the same time bending your knees. Return to the starting position, and repeat. Make sure your heels remain on the floor and keep your head up at all times. Keep good control throughout. Do 12.

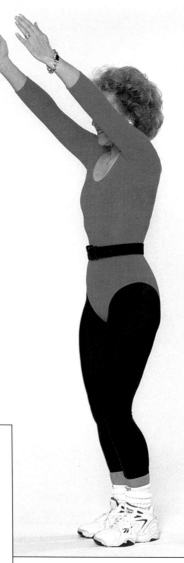

Kicks Out

Kick across with alternate legs, swinging your arms in the opposite direction. Keep your tummy pulled in and your shoulders back. Do 24.

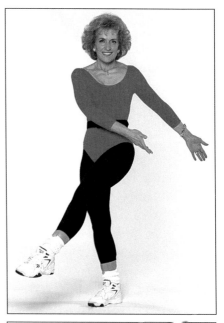

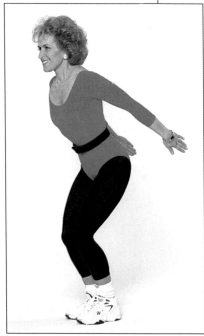

Kicks Back

Kick back with alternate feet, crossing your arms in front. Always maintain a slight bend in the supporting knee. Do 24.

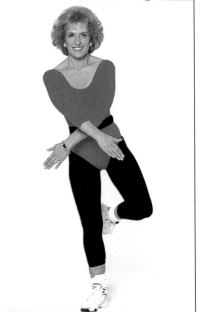

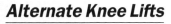

Alternate Knee Lifts

Raise alternate knees in front to waist level only, placing the opposite hand towards the raised knee. Keep your head up and take care not to lean forwards. Do 16.

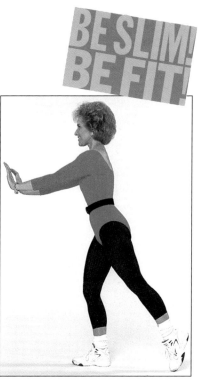

Push Backs

Take alternate legs behind you as you press your arms forwards. Keep your tummy tight and head up. Do 16.

Half Jacks

Push alternate feet out to the side, at the same time taking the arms out. Stand tall and keep the supporting knee bent. Do 16.

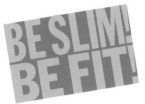
BE SLIM! BE FIT!

Curtsy Pecdecs

Take alternate legs diagonally behind you as if about to curtsy and, at the same time, draw your elbows in front of your chest. Do 16.

Lunges

As you push one leg out to the side and slightly to the back of you on a diagonal, push the same arm as leg across in the opposite direction. Control the move and keep your tummy tight. Repeat with the other arm and leg. Do 24.

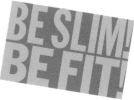

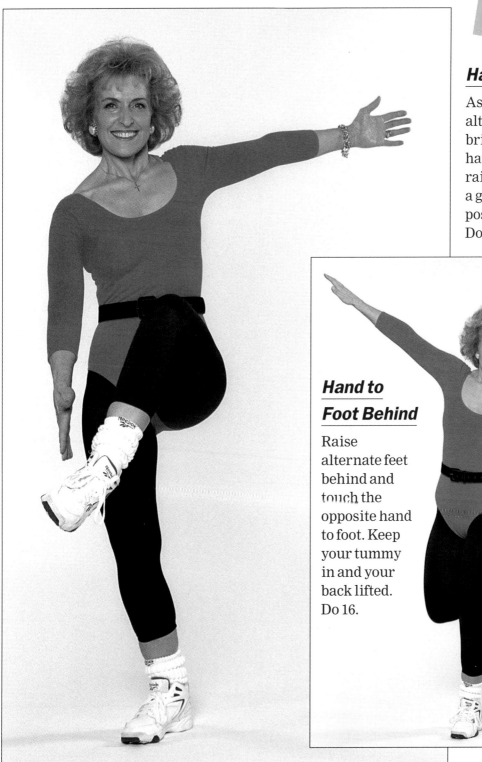

Hand to Foot

As you draw up alternate knees, bring the opposite hand towards the raised foot. Maintain a good, upright posture at all times. Do 16.

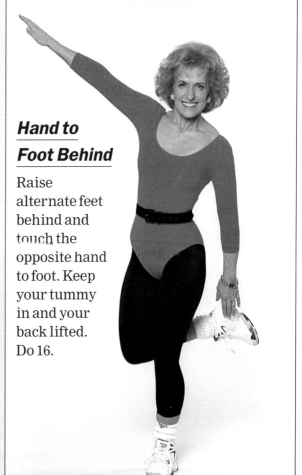

Hand to Foot Behind

Raise alternate feet behind and touch the opposite hand to foot. Keep your tummy in and your back lifted. Do 16.

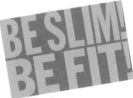

Toning for the Upper Body

Chest Shaper

Lie on the floor with knees bent. Place your arms on the floor, bent at a 90-degree angle, with elbows in line with your shoulders. Now raise the arms in front of the chest and squeeze the elbows towards each other. Do 16.

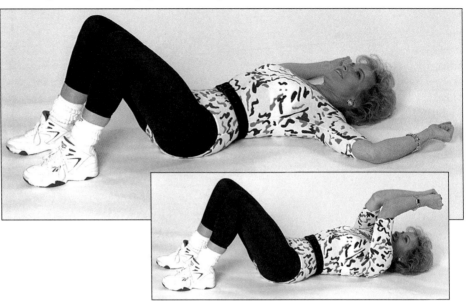

Press-ups for the Chest and Underarms

Position yourself on your hands and knees in a 'box shape', with hands under the shoulders and knees under the hips. Pull your tummy in tight to flatten your back. Now lower your forehead towards the floor in between your hands, pushing your elbows out to the sides. Press back up without locking your elbows.
Do 8, rest, then do 8 more.

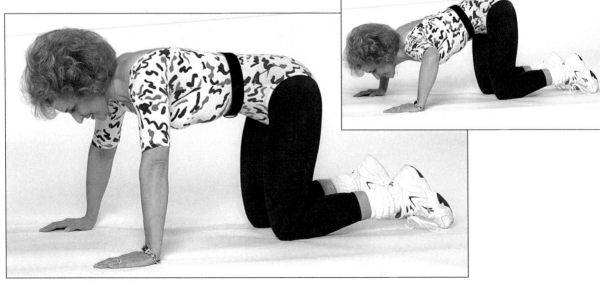

THE BE SLIM! BE FIT! EXERCISE PLAN

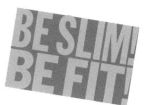

Upper Arm Shaper

Sit with legs comfortably crossed and your back lifted, and take your hands behind your hips, with elbows bent. Now, without dropping the level of the arms, extend the arms backwards. Do 8, rest, then do 8 more.

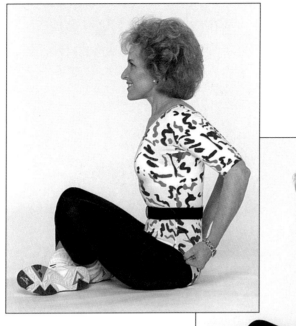

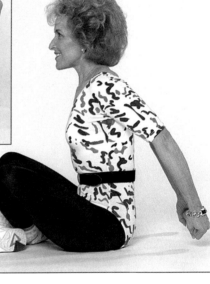

Upper Back Strengthener

Sit with legs comfortably crossed and your back straight. Place your arms at a 90-degree angle at shoulder height and squeeze the shoulders back. Do 6, rest, then do 6 more.

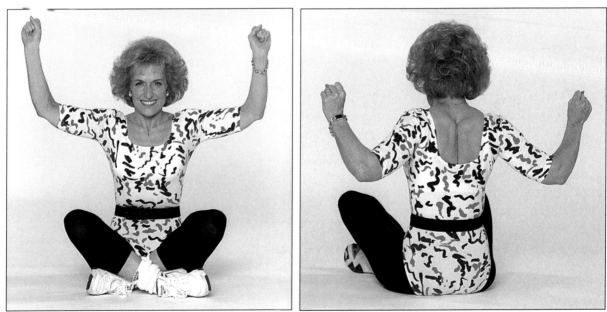

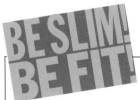

Advanced Upper Back Strengthener

Lie face down with arms bent at a 90-degree angle and elbows at shoulder height. Keep your head down and slowly lift your arms and shoulders off the floor. Do 6, rest, then do 6 more.

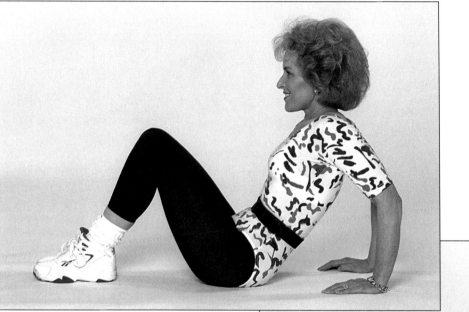

Advanced Upper Arm Shaper

Sit on the floor with arms bent and hands placed a comfortable distance behind you, fingers pointing towards your hips. Keeping both palms flat on the floor, bend from the elbows, then push firmly up again. Keep your tummy tight throughout. Do 6, rest, then do 6 more.

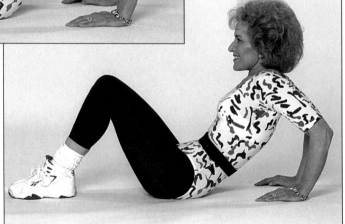

Toning for the Middle Body

Pelvic Tilt

Lie on the floor with knees bent. Pull your tummy in tight and press your lower back into the floor, raising your hips slightly. Breathe out as you press into the floor. Repeat 6–8 times.

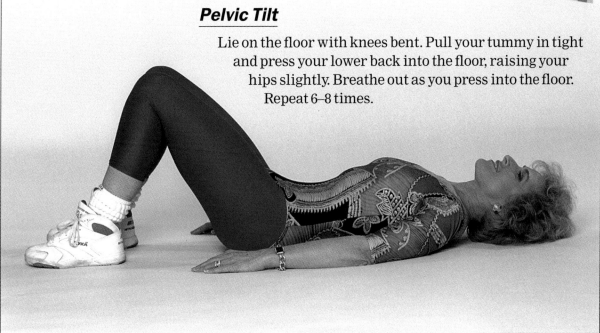

Tummy Toner

Pull your tummy in and gently raise your head and shoulders off the floor, sliding your hands up your thighs. Keep a distance between your chin and your chest. Slowly lower the head and shoulders to the floor. Do 6–8, breathing out as you lift and breathing in as you lower.

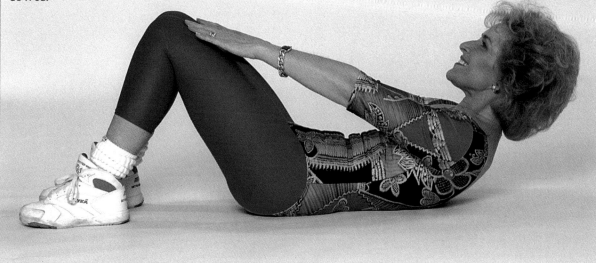

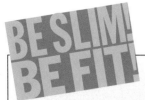

Advanced Tummy Toner

Place your hands to either side of your head. Keeping the elbows wide, raise your head and shoulders off the floor. Keep a distance between your chin and your chest as you raise. Slowly lower back down to the floor. Do 10–12, breathing out as you lift and breathing in as you lower.

Waist Trimmer

Place one hand behind your head. Keeping that elbow on the floor, reach the other hand towards the opposite knee. Keep your tummy tight and make a smooth lift. Return to to the floor and repeat to the other side. Breathe out as you lift and breathe in as you lower. Do 8, rest, then repeat.

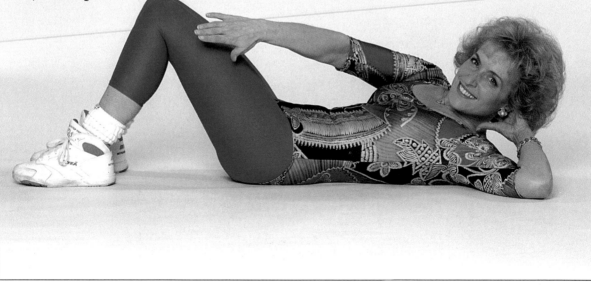

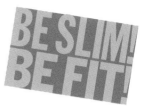

Advanced Waist Trimmer

Place your hands to either side of your head. Pull your tummy in tight and lift one shoulder off the floor towards the opposite knee. You don't need to lift too high. Slowly lower again, and repeat with the other shoulder to the opposite knee, breathing out as you lift and breathing in as you lower. Do 8, rest, then repeat.

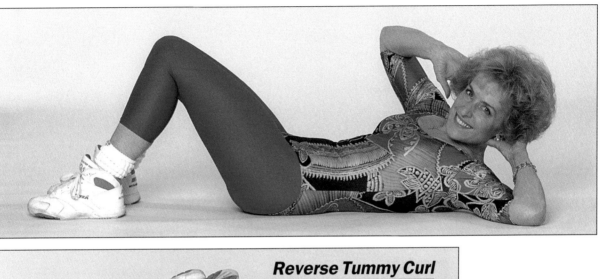

Reverse Tummy Curl

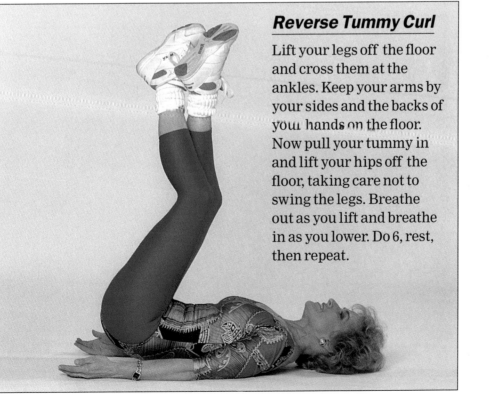

Lift your legs off the floor and cross them at the ankles. Keep your arms by your sides and the backs of your hands on the floor. Now pull your tummy in and lift your hips off the floor, taking care not to swing the legs. Breathe out as you lift and breathe in as you lower. Do 6, rest, then repeat.

Back Strengthener

Lie face down with elbows tucked in by your sides and palms facing up. Gently lift the upper body off the floor in a smooth action. Breathe out as you lift and breathe in as you lower. Do 6, rest, then repeat.

Advanced Back Strengthener

Lie face down with arms by your sides, palms facing up. Keeping your eyes looking at the floor and your feet firmly down, gently lift the upper body from the floor. Do 6, rest, then repeat.

Back Mobiliser

Come up on to your hands and knees, with hands placed under your shoulders and your knees placed under your hips. Pull your tummy in tight and lift your back up. Relax, and repeat 6–8 times.

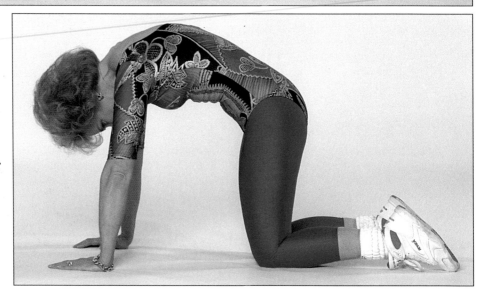

Toning for the Lower Body

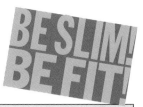

Outer Thigh Toner

Lie on your side with your head comfortably propped up on one hand. Bend the underneath leg and keep the top leg straight. Now lift the top leg, keeping the hips forwards and the leg in line with your trunk. Do 16, then roll over and repeat with the other leg.

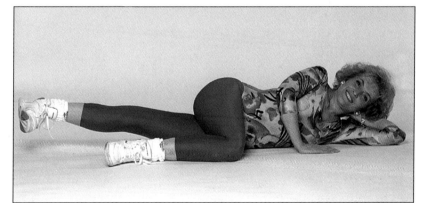

Inner Thigh Toner

Lie on your side with your head propped comfortably on your hand. Bend the top leg and bring the knee over to rest on the floor. Keep the underneath leg straight, and lift and lower it smoothly. Do 8, rest, then repeat. Roll over and repeat on the other side.

Advanced Inner Thigh Toner

Lie on your side and position the ankle of the top leg just above the knee of the underneath leg. Now lift the underneath leg in a slow and controlled manner. Do 12, rest, then repeat. Roll over and repeat on the other side.

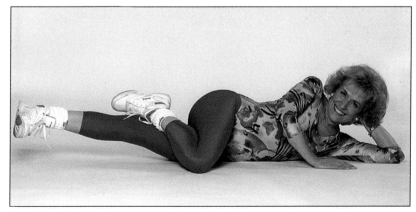

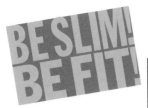

Bottom Shaper

Lie on your side with both knees slightly bent. Dip the knee of the top leg on the floor in front then, leading with the heel, extend and straighten the leg towards the back corner of the room. Try to make sure there is no movement in the spine, and keep the action smooth and controlled. Do 12, rest, then repeat. Roll over and repeat on the other side.

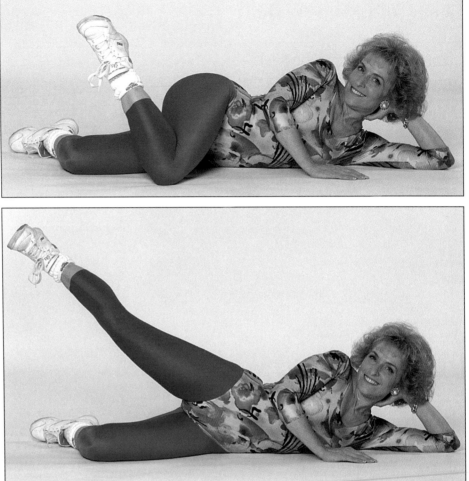

Bottom Toner

Lie face down with your head resting on your hands. Now lift one leg up, keeping the hips facing the floor. Bring the leg down again, and repeat with the other leg. Do 12, alternating legs.

Advanced Bottom Toner

Position yourself on your forearms and knees, then extend one leg
behind so that the toes rest on the floor. Now, keeping your tummy
tight and hips facing the floor, lift the extended leg, then lower it
again. There should be no movement in your spine.
Do 12–14, then change legs and repeat.

Back of Thigh Toner

Lie face down with your head resting on your hands. Cross your legs at
the ankles. Pressing your hips into the floor, bend the knees as you bring
your heels towards your seat. Do 12, then change legs and repeat with
the other leg on top.

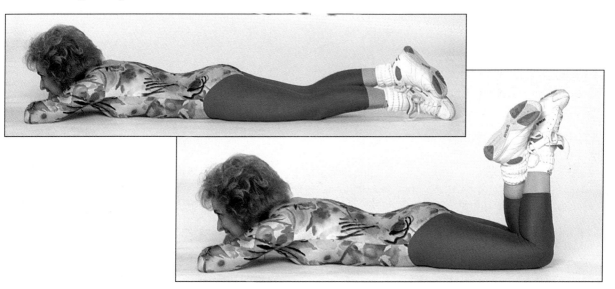

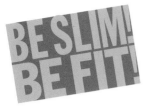

Front of Thigh Shaper

Prop yourself up on your elbows, keeping a distance between your head and your elbows. Bend one knee and place the foot flat on the floor. Extend the other leg away from the body with toes pulled towards you. Now lift and lower the straight leg, making sure the knee does not go beyond the level of the other knee. Keep the movement controlled. Do 16, then change legs and repeat.

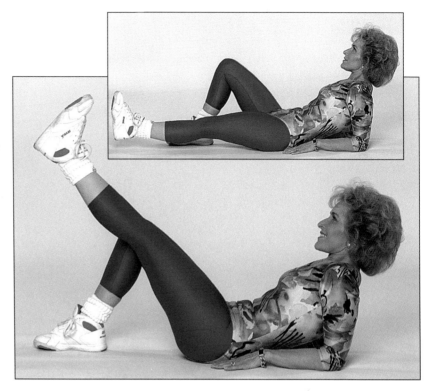

Bottom Toner

Lie on your back with knees bent and feet flat on the floor. Place your arms by your sides. Pull your tummy in tight and tilt the hips under slightly. Now, maintaining the hips in this position, lift them off the floor, squeezing the buttocks tightly, then release. Do 12, rest, then repeat.

Cool-down and Stretch

Chest Stretch

Sit with legs comfortably crossed and your back straight. Clasp your hands behind you and squeeze the shoulder blades together. Hold for 10 seconds, then release.

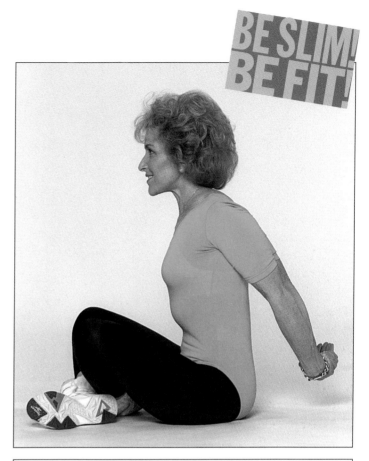

Upper Back Stretch

Sit with legs comfortably crossed. Pull your tummy in tight and take your arms out in front at chest height. Keeping your head down, press your upper back away from the hands and feel the shoulder blades pull further apart. Hold for 8–10 seconds, then release.

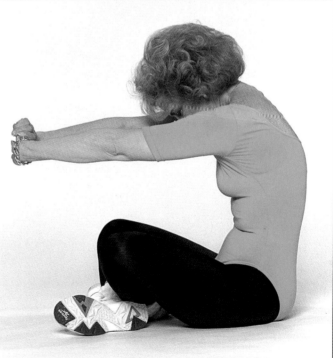

Outer Thigh and Waist Stretch

Sit with legs extended and take one leg across the other, placing the foot down in line with the other knee. Take the opposite arm across the bent leg and turn away from the leg. Use the other hand on the floor for support. Try to keep your back lifted. Hold for 8–10 seconds, then release. Change legs and repeat to the other side.

Inner Thigh Stretch

Sit up with soles of the feet together. Using your elbows, gently ease your knees down until you feel a stretch in the inside thighs. Hold for 15 seconds, then release.

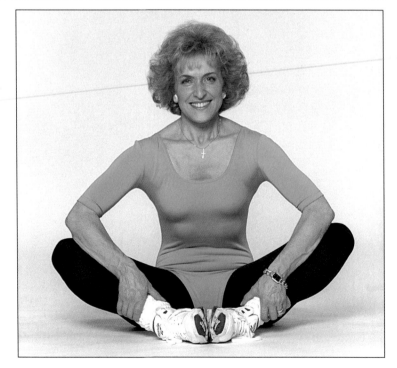

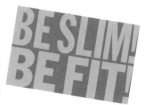

Back of Arm Stretch

Sit with legs comfortably crossed, head up and your back lifted. Place one hand behind your shoulder and use the other hand to press the arm further back until the elbow points towards the ceiling. Hold for 8–10 seconds, then release. Repeat to stretch out the other arm.

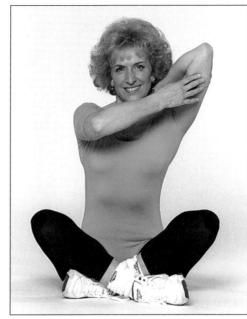

Back Stretch

Sit with legs crossed and hands on the floor in front of you. Lower your head then follow with the rest of the body until you feel a stretch down your spine. Hold for 8–10 seconds, then slowly come up.

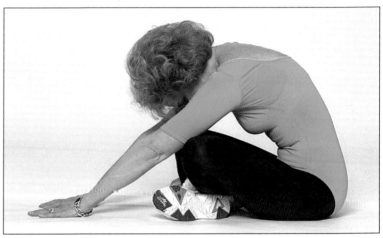

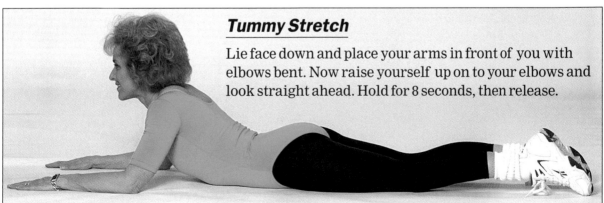

Tummy Stretch

Lie face down and place your arms in front of you with elbows bent. Now raise yourself up on to your elbows and look straight ahead. Hold for 8 seconds, then release.

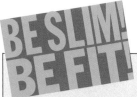

Front of Thigh Stretch

Lie face down with one hand resting under your chin. Take hold of one ankle with the other hand and gently press your hip to the floor. Hold for 8–10 seconds, then release. Repeat with the other leg.

Back of Thigh Stretch

Sit up with one leg extended and the other bent. Keep your hips secure on the floor and your back lifted as you take your trunk towards the extended leg. Hold for 15 seconds, then release. Change legs and repeat.

Full Body Stretch

Lie on your back. Take your arms over your head and gently
extend the whole body, pushing your hands as far away
from your feet as possible. Hold for 8 seconds,
then release.

Relax

Lie on your back with arms by your sides and legs extended. Try to
release the tension from the whole of your body. You deserve it.

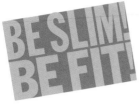

The Five-minute Workout
Warm-up

Shoulder Rolls

Roll alternate
shoulders
backwards,
transferring your
weight from one
foot to the other.
Hold your tummy
in and stand tall
throughout. Do 24.

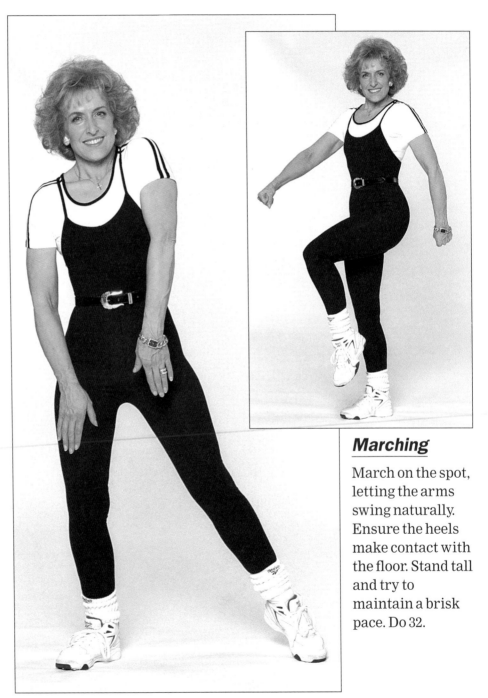

Marching

March on the spot,
letting the arms
swing naturally.
Ensure the heels
make contact with
the floor. Stand tall
and try to
maintain a brisk
pace. Do 32.

Knee Bends

Stand with feet wide apart and toes turned slightly out. Keep your back lifted as you bend from the knees and the hips as if about to sit in a chair. Ensure the knees bend outwards in line with the toes. Do 16.

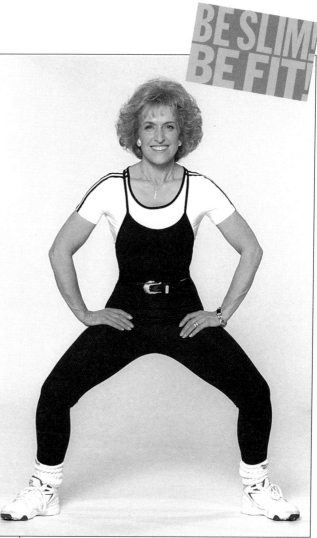

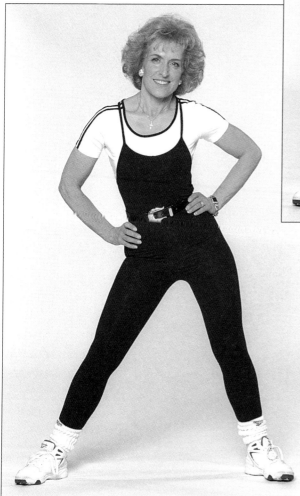

Hip Rolls

With knees slightly bent, rotate your hips. Do 8 in one direction, then repeat in the other direction.

Body Toning

Tummy Toner

Lie on your back with knees bent and feet flat on the floor. Place your hands on your thighs. Pull your tummy in tight and press your lower back into the floor. Lift the head and shoulders off the floor, sliding your hands up your thighs, then lower again. Breathe out as you lift and breathe in as you lower. Do 12.

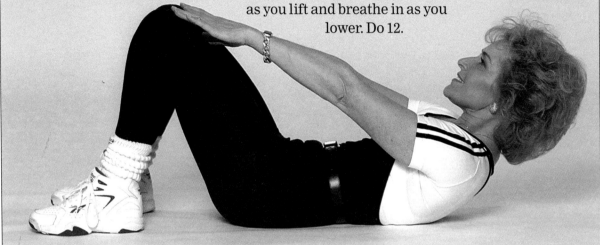

Outer Thigh Toner

Lie on your side with your head propped comfortably on your hand. Bend the underneath leg and keep the top leg straight. Now lift the top leg, keeping the hips forwards and the leg in line with the trunk. Do 16, then roll over and repeat with the other leg.

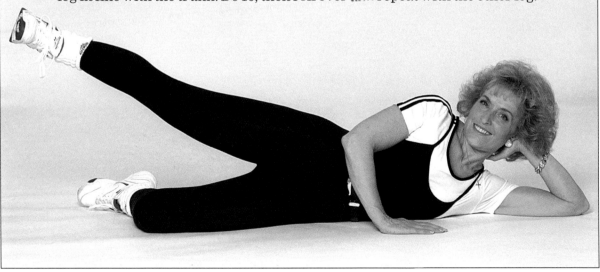

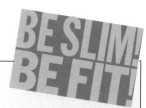

Inner Thigh Toner

Lie on your side with your head propped comfortably on your hand. Take the top leg over in front and rest the knee on the floor. Straighten the underneath leg and lift it up and down smoothly. Do 8, rest, then repeat. Roll over and repeat with the other leg.

Back Strengthener

Lie face down with elbows tucked in by your sides and hands crossed on your seat with palms facing up. Gently lift your upper body from the floor in a smooth action. Breathe out as you lift and breathe in as you lower. Do 6, rest, then repeat.

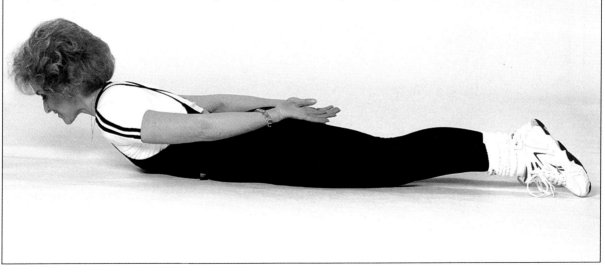

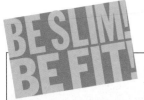

Chest and Underarm Toner

Position yourself on your hands and knees, making a 'box' shape, with hands under your shoulders and knees under your hips. Pull your tummy in tight to flatten your back. Now lower your forehead down in between your hands, pushing the elbows out. Press back up without locking your elbows. Do 8, rest, then do 8 more.

Waist Trimmer

Lie on your back and place one hand behind your head. Keeping that elbow on the floor, reach the other hand towards the opposite knee. Keep your tummy in tight and make a smooth lift. Return to the floor and repeat to the other side. Do 8 to alternate sides, rest, then do 8 more.

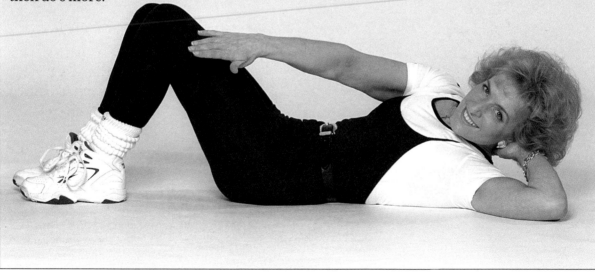

Cool-down and Stretch

Back of Thigh Stretch

Lie on your back with knees bent. Take hold of one leg, placing one hand at the back of the thigh and the other hand at the back of the calf, and squeeze the leg towards your chest. Now extend the lower leg until you feel tension in the back of the thigh of the raised leg. Keep both hips on the floor and keep your neck and shoulders relaxed. Hold for 10 seconds, release, then pull the leg towards your chest again for a further 10 seconds. Repeat with the other leg.

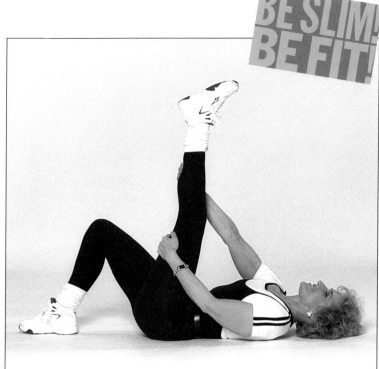

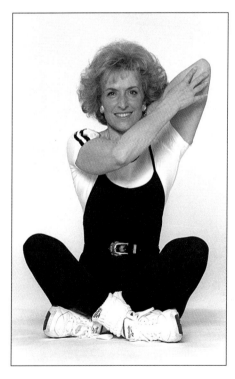

Back of Arm Stretch

Sit with legs comfortably crossed and your back lifted, head up. Place one hand behind the shoulder and use the other hand to press the arm further back until the elbow points to the ceiling. Hold for 8–10 seconds, then change arms and repeat.

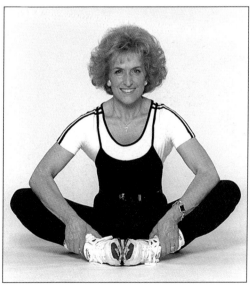

Inner Thigh Stretch

Sit up with soles of the feet together. Using your elbows, gently ease your knees down until you feel the stretch in the inside thighs. Hold for 15 seconds, then release.

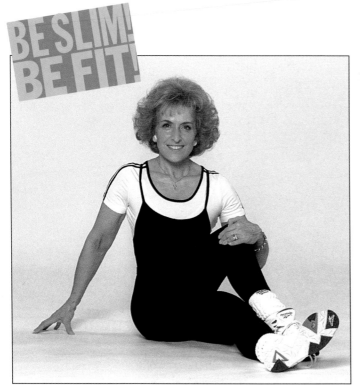

Outer Thigh Stretch

Sit up with legs extended in front. Cross one leg over the other leg and place the foot level with the knee. Place the hand on the same side on the floor for support. Place the other hand at the outside of the bent knee and gently pull the knee across the body. Hold for 8–10 seconds, then change legs and repeat.

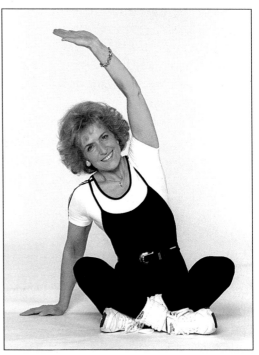

Chest Stretch

Sit with legs comfortably crossed and your back straight. Clasp your hands behind you and squeeze your shoulder blades together. Hold for 10 seconds, then release.

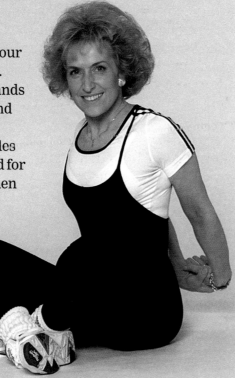

Waist Stretch

Sit with legs comfortably crossed and your back straight. Take one arm up above your head and lift up towards the ceiling. Now gently lean towards the arm on the floor until you feel the stretch in your waist. Keep both hips on the floor at all times and try not to lean forwards or back. Hold for 8–10 seconds, then repeat to the other side.

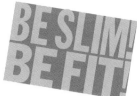

Be Slim! Be Fit! For Life

You should now be well into the swing of low-fat eating and increased activity, and the good habits that you have acquired during your Be Slim! Be Fit! campaign will stand you in good stead for life. So once you have reached your desired weight, don't give up! Eating healthily and keeping active will pay enormous dividends, not just in terms of your weight and body shape but also in terms of your overall health and wellbeing.

However, you can now relax the rules a little and increase the quantities of food you eat. You may add a few more dressings to salads and eat a little low-fat hard cheese, but if you are to maintain your new-found figure and energy you will still need to follow a low-fat formula and take regular exercise. We only regain weight if we go back to our old, bad habits. So continue to eat low fat and try to exercise at least three times a week for at least 20 minutes each time.

The good news is that our tastebuds adapt – for many the taste of fatty food becomes repulsive – and so it is relatively simple to stick with our new low-fat way of eating and keep the excess weight off for good. And once we are used to a regular programme of activity, we feel so good that we *want* to keep it up.

Keep an eye on the scales and the tape measure. It you find you are gaining weight again, return to the diet or cut back on the quantities. If you take immediate action, you can remedy any damage quite swiftly.

When dining out, select carefully from the menu. By all means eat the bread roll, but try to refrain from putting butter on it. Choose a light fat-free starter such as melon. For your main course, have fish or chicken cooked without fat and ask for vegetables to be served without butter. Select a dessert that is fruit or sorbet (Pavlova is also fine if you have the willpower to leave the cream!) and avoid the cheeseboard at all costs. Drink sparkling mineral water alongside your wine as this will help fill you up. But most of all, enjoy it!

Remember, eating should be a pleasurable experience, and by following my Be Slim! Be Fit! philosophy you should still be able to eat well and heartily and feel better for it.

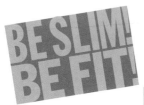

Here are my ten tips for weight maintenance.

Ten Tips For Weight Maintenance

1 Eat three meals a day and eat low-fat, high-volume foods. Not only will these fill you up, they will cause the body to work harder and burn more calories during the digestion process.

2 Always remember that the fat we eat becomes fat on our bodies. If we want to stay lean we have to eat lean. Use the Traffic Light Guide on pages 25 to 28 for a quick and easy check on which foods to eat and which to avoid.

3 Do not eat between meals – nibbling between meals can seriously damage your waistline.

4 Avoid temptation by not keeping biscuits and sweets in the house. Instead, have plenty of fresh fruit available and keep the refrigerator stocked with diet drinks and diet yogurts to satisfy sweet cravings.

5 Never skip a meal, since this can lead to uncontrolled eating later, and always eat breakfast to help kick-start your metabolism each day.

6 The occasional indiscretion is not the end of the world, but do remember that one lapse can lead to another, so indulge with caution!

7 Continue to be as physically active as possible. Aerobic exercise will keep your heart fitter and also keep your metabolic rate higher so that weight maintenance becomes easy.

8 Exercise should always be enjoyable. Try to vary your activities so that you don't get bored.

9 Don't forget to practise good posture habits at all times throughout the day. Good posture will keep you looking slimmer and younger.

10 Remember that *you* are in control of your body and your lifestyle. If you want to stay slim and fit, you *can* do so.

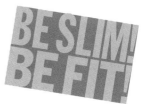
BE SLIM!
BE FIT!

Making the Most of Yourself

Through healthy eating and regular exercise we can make incredible improvements to our body shape. But the way we carry and dress ourselves also affects the way we look. Dressing carefully can maximise our best features and at the same time minimise those areas we want to play down. By practising good posture habits and choosing clothes wisely we can significantly enhance our appearance.

Generally, we fall into three basic body shapes. We tend to be either pear-shaped, apple-shaped or heart-shaped. We can't change the basic shape that Nature gave us, but whatever shape or size we are, we can make the best of what we've got. The style of our clothes can have the effect of making us look pounds heavier or lighter than we really are. Here are some tips to help you create your most flattering look.

First we need to get our underwear right. A badly-fitting bra or the unsightly outline of a pair of skimpy panties cutting into an over-ample posterior can kill the look of a beautiful dress.

Whether you are well endowed or relatively small-chested, a well-fitting bra will dramatically enhance your figure. Few people know how to measure themselves for a bra and feel embarrassed to ask for help when choosing one. Most women select them on a trial-and-error basis and hope that after a couple of washes it will mould to their shape!

Measuring yourself for a bra is really easy. First, measure around the area just below your bust (as high as possible without including the breasts). If the measurement is even, add four inches (10 cm); if it is odd, add five inches (12.5 cm). This will give you your bra size.

To find your cup size, measure around the fullest part of your bust (wearing a bra). If that measurement is the same as the first measurement (including the additional four or five inches) you need an A cup. If it is one inch (2.5 cm) larger you need a B cup, two inches (5 cm) larger, a C cup – and so on. Always try on a bra before buying it. It shouldn't cut into your shoulders or your back and you should not bulge out at the top of the cups.

Because flesh and fat are moveable, our underwear often has the effect of creating bulges if we wear the same styles all the time. Check if

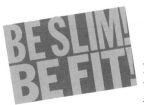

you have wedges of fat on your back, over and under your bra – and whether you have saddlebags above your pants. If you do, you should vary the styles you choose so that the fat does not settle in one spot.

Bikini briefs may look pretty, but they often dig in and create unsightly bulges which, over a period of time, become permanent. Try to wear a different style of briefs each day – some high-cut, some low-cut. And make sure they fit fairly loosely. Go for the next size if necessary.

Wearing a correctly-fitting bra and having a smooth contour around your hips will not only give you a more attractive appearance, it will make you look slimmer too.

The Pear Shape

If you have hefty hips, jodhpur thighs, a big bottom but a proportionately slim waist, then you are pear-shaped. Here are my ten tips for a more streamlined look:

Ten Tips For Pear Shapes

1 Wear darker colours below the waist and lighter colours above.
2 Wear plain colours below the waist and patterns above.
3 Avoid pleated skirts and slacks with pleat tucks into the waistline.
4 Wear long skirts that will make you look slimmer and avoid short ones which will have the reverse effect.
5 Colour co-ordinate your tights with your skirt to avoid 'breaking up' the overall look – navy tights with a navy skirt, black with black etc. – and make sure your shoes match too.
6 Pay attention to detail above the waist. Go for eye-catching blouses and waistcoats and jazzy jewellery.
7 Wear either long jackets that skim over the hips and thighs or really short ones that stop at the waist. Avoid those that finish on your widest part.
8 Show off your waistline with buckles and belts.
9 Wear high heels. Stilettos are back in fashion, so make the most of them and stand tall and slim.
10 Avoid leggings since these will not create the most flattering look for you.

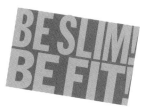

The Apple Shape

Characteristics of the apple shape are slim limbs, little or no waistline, a flattish bottom and a large tummy. If you fall into this category, make the most of those slim arms and legs that pear shapes would die for, and minimise attention on your middle area. Apple shapes are easy to flatter, so have some fun trying out different styles.

Ten Tips For Apple Shapes

1. Wear styles that skim over the waist such as blousons or tunics.
2. Wear dark colours over your torso, and choose trousers and skirts in pale colours or patterns to make you look stunning.
3. Avoid anything that is belted or draws attention to the waistline.
4. Wear blouses designed to sit outside your skirt.
5. Wear jackets loose enough and long enough to cover an ample tum but short enough to show off those thighs.
6. You'll look great in short sleeves and straps that show off your arms.
7. Wear pretty jewellery to attract attention above the waist.
8. Always ensure skirts and trousers are a comfortable fit. You'll look slimmer in clothes that don't cling.
9. Only wear skirts with pleats if the pleats start from below your hips and are sewn down over the tummy.
10. Show off your legs with loggings, and pair up with a stunning tabard top.

The Heart Shape

Characteristics of the heart shape are slim arms and legs, narrow hips and a large bust. Few women are happy with the size of their bust. We either have too little or too much. There is no point in trying to hide a large bust, but you can certainly keep it under proper control. There is no known exercise that will specifically reduce the breasts. Aerobic exercise is the only way to burn fat off the body, wherever the fat may be stored. Some sports shops stock a special 'Aero bra' which has been designed to give extra support during exercise.

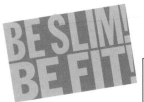

Ten Tips For Heart Shapes

1 Wear dark colours above the waist to detract from the bust area.

2 Show off your slim hips and thighs with light-coloured skirts and trousers.

3 Keep blouses plain – without frills or patterns.

4 Pleated skirts and trousers look great on heart shapes.

5 Shoulder pads will give your appearance a crisper look and will help balance the upper body.

6 A good, well-supporting bra is essential and this may require professional fitting.

7 Pay particular attention to shoes, tights and skirt length. You most likely have stunning legs, so make the most of them.

8 Beware of wearing high heels with a short skirt as this will not create the most flattering combination for you.

9 Choose jewellery carefully and avoid drop earrings and long ropes of beads. You need jewellery that will attract the eye upwards, not downwards.

10 Cross-over styles of dresses and tops will suit you well but avoid plunge necklines.

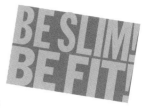
BE SLIM!
BE FIT!

Over the years I have received many letters from slimmers with a variety of questions about diet and exercise. In this chapter I have included a selection of questions which high-light some of the most common dieting or exercise problems.

Your Questions Answered

Diet

Q I can go all day without food and I only eat one meal in the evening, so why am I overweight?

A Going without food like that is the worst thing you can do when you are trying to lose weight. You need to eat three meals a day at regular intervals to keep your metabolic rate buoyant. Eating one meal a day sends messages to your body saying: 'Starvation!' So it stores the food you give it once a day as fat, in case of emergencies, rather than providing you with the energy you need. It is particularly important to eat breakfast, and I also suggest you try eating fruit for lunch since it is a quick and easy option as well as being nutritious.

Q Most diets stipulate that you must eat breakfast, but I just can't face it. I want to lose weight, and won't I actually lose more weight if I skip this meal?

A We need to eat breakfast to kick-start our metabolism first thing in the morning. In fact, if you skip it you will lose less weight, not more!

If you really can't eat first thing, have a glass of unsweetened orange juice ($1/4$ pint/125 ml) when you get up and take some fruit to work to eat mid-morning. This will help you on your way.

Q Last year I went on a meal replacement diet and lost three stone (19 kg). Then I stopped and I have since regained all the weight I lost plus two more stone (12.7 kg)! I am desperate. Please help me.

A Anyone who follows a very-low-calorie diet such as you describe will find that it has the effect of slowing down the metabolic rate, since the body holds on to the food we do eat in case we stop eating altogether. By crash dieting you will have lost some muscle mass, which means that your body now needs less calories to sustain it. Remember, the more muscle mass we have, the more calories we will burn.

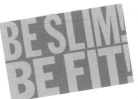

In your case you need to eat six small meals a day totalling around 1,500 calories of low-fat food, and you need to increase the amount of exercise you take so that you can build up your energy output to help you burn more fat. It will take time, but with patience and sensible eating you can succeed.

Q I have a slow metabolism as a result of crash dieting. Is there anything at all I can do to help speed it up and lose some of my ugly fat?

A We can speed up our metabolic rate in a variety of ways. First, resolve NEVER to crash diet again. Instead, eat three low-fat, high nutrition meals a day and to help your body realise that it isn't going to be starved. Next, try to be as physically active as possible and include some toning exercises, since these will help build more muscle. The more muscle mass we have, the higher our metabolic rate.

Q I have lost four stone (25.4 kg) in six months on a diet, but my weight has not moved for the past five weeks. I am sticking to the diet and I exercise regularly as I still have more weight to lose. What else can I do?

A Well done for losing so much weight so far. Your body has now become acclimatised to having less food than it used to have and needs to be persuaded that you are not dieting! Try eating a little more each day – perhaps two extra pieces of fruit or an extra slice of bread – and also step up the daily exercise. After a fortnight, go back to the diet and watch the last few pounds drop away. Keep up the increased level of exercise as this will help keep your metabolic rate from falling again.

Q I have been on your diet and exercise programme for four months. My original weight was ten stone three pounds (64.9 kg) and I am now eight stone five pounds (53 kg). However, my target weight is eight stone (51 kg). I have remained the same weight now for three weeks and appear to be stuck! Have you any suggestions?

A Congratulations on doing well so far. The last few pounds are always the hardest to shift. You need to persuade your body it's not on a diet. Increase your food portions by ten per cent for two weeks, and increase the amount of aerobic exercise by five minutes a day. Then continue with the exercises but return to the diet and watch those last few pounds disappear!

Q I have one and a half stone (9.5 kg) to lose, but I am finding it impossible. I'm on a very-low-calorie, low-fat diet of 700 to 800 calories per day, and I take regular exercise. Do I have to eat even fewer calories to lose weight?

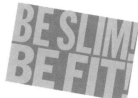

A No. You must increase your calorie intake because you are not giving your body sufficient food to function properly. Gradually increase your calorie intake by adding an extra 200 calories a day for week one, then another 200 for weeks two and three. Continue like this until you are eating around 1,400–1,500 calories per day. Eat healthy, low-fat food and keep exercising. You will then start to lose weight. You will be amazed how much more you'll lose when you eat properly.

Q I am desperate to lose two stone (12.7 kg) but I am a chocoholic. What can I do?

A Chocolate is full of fat, which turns to fat on your body when you eat it. If you want to have a lean body you must decide to give up the chocolate. Set yourself short-term goals, such as going three days without it, and then see if you can go another day, and so on. If you have to give in to your craving, limit the amount to one small bar, and then try again with another goal and see how long you can abstain. What you must NOT do is feel that when you have your first cheat the whole campaign is ruined, and then eat six bars! If you want to be slim badly enough you can give up the chocolate – and if you can go without it for 30 days you will have broken the habit.

Q I just adore chips but I know I need to lose weight. Can you suggest anything?

A You can make fat-free oven chips yourself. Peel and chop a large potato into chips. Place the uncooked chips into boiling water with a stock cube and cook for two minutes. Remove the chips from the stock and place them on a hot baking tray. Sprinkle with salt, then place them on the top shelf of a hot oven (200°C, 400°F, or Gas Mark 6) and cook until golden brown (about 30 minutes). Turn them over during cooking to ensure they brown evenly.

Q My husband needs to lose weight but won't go on a diet. It really worries me because his father died of a heart attack two years ago. What can I do?

A By selecting low-fat food and cooking without fat you can put your husband on a low-fat diet and he won't even notice.
Serve him low-fat rice dishes instead of chips, and healthy low-fat desserts instead of stodgy high-fat puddings. With a little time and imagination you can spoil him with delicious low-fat goodies.

Q My husband and I are retired and enjoy our main meal at lunchtime. We both need to lose about one and a half stone (9.5 kg), but most diets include the main meal in the evening. Do we have to eat then?

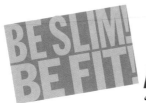

A Not at all. The earlier in the day you eat your main meal, the more chance you have to work off the calories. You've heard the saying: 'Breakfast like a king, lunch like a prince and dine like a pauper.' Well, ideally that IS best, but most people's lifestyles aren't able to cope with this pattern because of their work schedules.

But you CAN make these choices, so just swap round the lunch and dinner menus and enjoy yourselves.

Q Because of my lifestyle I have to eat late at night. Is this why I can't lose weight?

A It is more likely to be WHAT you eat rather than when you eat it that is the problem. It is preferable to eat earlier in the evening because we don't sleep so well on a full stomach and the earlier we eat, the more chance we have to work off the calories. If you are eating later, try to have a lighter meal and perhaps arrange to have a more substantial lunch. But do check WHAT you eat and eat only low-fat foods.

Q I have three children and now find I am expecting my fourth! With each of the others I gained three stone (19 kg) and getting the weight off again afterwards proved increasingly difficult. Any suggestions to prevent so much weight gain this time?

A Well done for taking steps to keep your weight under control during this pregnancy. Eat plenty of low-fat, high nutritious foods, such as lean meat, poultry and fish and loads of vegetables, fruit and salads.

Each day drink $1/2$ to $3/4$ pint (250–375 ml) of semi-skimmed milk and include bread, potatoes, cereal, rice and pasta in your diet too.

Don't snack on biscuits, cakes, sweets, since these will just turn to fat on your body. Be as physically active as possible and DON'T eat for two! Also, remember to avoid soft cheese and liver throughout the pregnancy.

Q My daughter is 17 and just seems to be gaining more weight. The more I moan at her, the more she seems to eat. What can I do?

A Leave her alone. Your daughter is reacting to your pressure and it's having the opposite affect. As she gets older she will decide to slim down when SHE wants to. You can help by preparing healthy, nutritious meals and by encouraging her to take more exercise. You could also offer support by going with her to a local fitness class.

Q I am going on holiday in six weeks' time. How can I lose two stone (12.7 kg) quickly?

A Between now and your holiday you could lose one stone (6.4 kg) if you stick rigidly to a low-fat diet, and you'll feel much better. If you eat sensibly while you are away and are as physically active as possible,

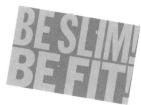

you will keep your metabolic rate buoyant so that when you get home you can continue on the low-fat diet and lose the remaining stone. You CAN do it. Start today, eat sensibly and take lots of exercise. You'll be thrilled with the results.

Q I hate yogurt and fromage frais, but they seem to be included in every diet I try. What can I eat instead so that I don't lose out nutritionally?

A Both are rich sources of calcium, which is important in our daily diet, so I suggest you increase your daily milk allowance from $1/_2$ pint (250 ml) to $3/_4$ pint (375 ml) to compensate.

Q I don't have time to make sandwiches for lunch. What can I try instead?

A Try a Golden Wonder 'Pot Light' or a Heinz 'Lunch Bowl', plus a piece of fruit or yogurt. Allow yourself approximately 300 calories and vary your choices. Fruit, yogurt, slimmers' cup a soups and fresh wholemeal bread are also quick and easy options.

Q I got into great shape for my holiday, and it was wonderful. Now I'm back and discover I have gained eight pounds (3.6 kg)! What can I do?

A Weight gained quickly can be lost quickly too. The secret is to take immediate action. Go back on a low-fat diet, don't cheat at all, and exercise as much as possible. You'll be surprised how quickly that holiday weight will disappear.

Q What is your view on food combining? Would it help me to lose weight more quickly?

A I don't believe it has any magical qualities to help or speed up weight loss. Since you are not allowed to combine certain food groups at the same meal, the calorie consumption is automatically reduced. However, I feel it is unnatural and impractical. There are easier ways to lose weight and keep it off.

Q Whenever I have dieted before I have always lost weight from the places where I've wanted to keep it, particularly from my bust. What steps can I take to prevent this?

A We all store fat in different places, depending on whether we are pear-, apple- or heart-shaped. In my experience if you follow a low-fat diet, you will find that you lose most fat from the fattest areas first, whereas on a calorie-controlled diet that still includes fat, you will lose it from those areas where you want to keep it. This is because you are still depositing fat into your body's bank account of fat, wherever these deposit boxes might be!

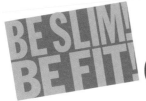

Q Is there such a thing as a good calorie?
Or are all calories the same?

A A calorie is a unit of energy, and calories are used to calculate the energy value of foods. Some foods such as sweets and alcohol contain what are often termed 'empty' calories, because they contribute few valuable nutrients. It obviously makes sense to eat calories from foods that help us become healthier by supplying essential nutrients such as protein, complex carbohydrates (starchy foods), vitamins and minerals.

Q Sweets contain hardly any fat.
Can I eat these on your low-fat diet?

A While sweets contain little fat, they are considered 'empty calories' since there are few nutrients in confectionery. If you eat sweets as well as your full quota from the diet menus you will of course be consuming more calories than you should and your weight-loss progress will slow down accordingly.

Sugar-free chewing gum is a good alternative, or you could treat yourself to a tube of Polos per week and see how long you can make them last.

Another alternative is to have a few sweets and compensate for the additional calories by doing more exercise. You could burn off the calories from a small packet of wine gums by doing 20 minutes' brisk walking! But if you do the walking and forget the wine gums, think how much more weight you will lose!

Q I understand that alcohol is allowed on your diets. But wouldn't I lose weight more quickly if I avoided alcohol altogether?

A Alcohol is allowed in moderation in my diets – one drink a day for women and two for men. Dieters often find that having a drink at the end of the day is something to look forward to – a treat in fact – and psychologically important in helping them stick to the diet. In turn, this leads to greater long-term success. But, beware! Too much alcohol will effectively reduce your willpower and can be harmful to health. If you don't like alcohol you can drink extra fruit juice.

Q I am three stone (19 kg) overweight and a diet failure. I can't afford to buy diet food and I can't exercise because I only have one lung. I do hope you can give me some hope and advice.

A Low-fat foods are no more expensive than high-fat foods – and you'll save money by not buying certain foods such as butter and oil. Bread, potatoes, fruit and vegetables, cereal, rice and pasta are all inexpensive foods and important for good nutrition. Eat fish or poultry (without the

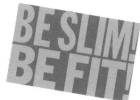

skin) in preference to red meat, and include foods like baked beans and chickpeas. You need to eat some low-fat dairy foods too, such as semi-skimmed milk and yogurt and cottage cheese. Try to eat three meals a day incorporating a variety of foods and always cook without fat. As you lose some weight you will be able to be a little more active. Walking is a really good way of exercising and should work for you.

Q I am going on a coaching holiday next month. It is half board and we will have lunch out on our touring days. Can you give me some tips for the lunches?

A Stick to the low-fat rule. Eat a jacket potato topped with cottage cheese or baked beans and served with salad, or eat any meat or poultry salad. If you choose sandwiches, ask for them to be prepared without butter and spread with horseradish sauce or pickle to add moisture and flavour. Avoid the ploughman's lunch and the chips, and you'll be fine. Have a great time.

Q I am a vegetarian and follow a low-fat diet. I see Quorn advertised as a vegetarian food. Is it low in fat?

A Yes, it is. It is rich in protein and should always be served in a sauce as, on its own, it doesn't have much flavour.

Q Is it necessary always to buy diet products such as low-sugar baked beans, jams and marmalades?

A The small amount of sugar found in regular baked beans should not hinder your chances of losing weight, and the regular brands are cheaper. Ordinary jams and marmalades taste infinitely better than the low-sugar brands, and my view is that the more 'normally' we eat and the fewer special foods we have to buy, the less likely we are to cheat because we won't feel deprived. However, choosing low-fat alternatives will greatly enhance your chances of success in losing weight. Fat contains more than twice as many calories as sugar and is more likely to be deposited as fat on your body.

Q I am just starting out on your diet. How much weight should I lose each week?

A It is impossible to predict any individual's rate of weight loss as we are all different, but if you follow any of my low-fat diets, you should lose $1\frac{1}{2}$ lb to 2 lb (0.7–0.9 kg) of fat from your body each week.

I emphasise 'fat loss' rather than 'weight loss' because it is inches you really want to shed. Don't be tempted by the 'quick-fix' meal replacement drinks which will cause you to lose mostly fluid and lean muscle tissue rather than fat.

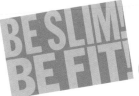

Q I drink lots of cups of tea in a day. Is that fattening?

A Black tea and coffee contain virtually no calories, so they can be drunk freely on a diet. However, if you include milk, that adds about 20 calories a cup. Add 20 calories more for each teaspoonful of sugar and that's where the calories can mount up. Any fluid we drink is processed by the body and eventually passes through us. However, it's not a good idea to drink tea or coffee in excess because of their caffeine content and the fact that they are dehydrating, which can cause mood swings and headaches. Try cutting down on the tea and coffee and increasing your intake of water – still or sparkling water is fine.

Q I am 61 years old, and in the past few months have gained a big spare tyre. I am dieting a bit and do a few exercises. Please tell me how I can get rid of it in time for my holiday.

A Your spare tyre has appeared because you have gained weight. 'Dieting a bit' is not helping you at all. It requires a total, determined effort if you are to succeed. Follow a low-fat diet and eat three meals a day, eating nothing in between meals. Fill up on vegetables and avoid all biscuits, chocolates, cakes and fried foods.

Q I have been on your low-fat diet for several months with great success. I have never felt better, but if I eat fatty food when dining out I feel quite ill with indigestion. Why?

A Your body has become used to eating healthily and likes it, which is why you feel so well. High-fat food is very indigestible and when you re-introduce it, your body protests. Don't worry – it will just encourage you to eat low fat, and that's good news.

Q I have been on a low-fat diet for some time. I now find I am pregnant. Can I stay on the diet? I hope so because I look and feel so much better than I used to.

A Yes, you can, but it is always a good idea to check with your doctor, since he will know your medical history. Eat lots of healthy foods – fruit, vegetables, lean meat and poultry – and avoid high-fat biscuits, cakes and chocolates. Try to be physically active too. Swimming is ideal.

Q I have been a yo-yo dieter for a while. Sometimes I eat once a day and just fill up on tea. Can you please help me to follow a proper diet?

A Yo-yo dieters, or people who binge then starve, find themselves in a worrying cycle with little confidence in their eating habits. If you follow the meal suggestions in this book and eat three meals a day, you will soon get into a proper routine again.

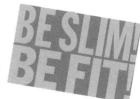

Q I am on a low-fat diet but I do use a little oil in my cooking. Will that affect the diet?

A Yes, it certainly will. Oil is 100 per cent fat, and you don't really need to use it in your cooking if you use non-stick pans. Try cooking with wines or low-fat sauces to add moisture and taste. By kicking the habit of adding oil, you will be amazed how much more quickly you'll lose your excess weight.

Q I have been following your low-fat diet for many months and feel so much better and have more energy. I never want to return to my old eating habits. Can I eat low-fat food for ever?

A Yes. A low-fat diet is a very healthy diet, providing you eat a variety of foods and include some oily fish such as tuna, mackerel or salmon. These contain vital nutrients, which are essential for good health. Well done for changing your unhealthy eating habits for the better. Continue to reap the rewards.

Q I really hate the taste of skimmed milk, but I am anxious to follow your diet. Is there an alternative?

A I can't bear skimmed milk either, but I find that semi-skimmed is infinitely more palatable. It is still low in fat and can work very well within a low-fat diet. Even though semi-skimmed milk contains a few more calories than skimmed milk, these extra calories are not sufficient to make a difference to your overall diet. Semi-skimmed milk also contains more calcium than whole milk, and you should aim to drink 1/2 pint (250 ml) a day.

Q I am sticking to your diet and I have lost loads of inches but not many pounds. Why is this?

A No two people are the same. Some people lose more weight than inches, while others lose more inches than pounds. There is no simple answer, but losing inches is what it's really about. If you are getting leaner and smaller, it doesn't really matter what you weigh. It's the fat that is disappearing, and that's terrific news.

Q I can't eat dairy products such as milk, yogurt and cottage cheese. Does it matter if I leave these out of my diet?

A All these foods are rich in nutrients and are particularly high in calcium and protein. If you are a meat-eater or eat lots of beans and pulses you are unlikely to be deficient in protein. Try soya milk and eat lots of green leafy vegetables, which contain calcium. It may also be necessary for you to take a calcium supplement. Your doctor or pharmacist should be able to recommend a suitable one.

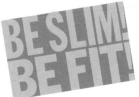

Q I have always taken cod liver oil capsules every day. I have just started on your low-fat diet, so will they still work for me?

A Yes, providing you don't take loads of them. One a day is fine. Oil is 100 per cent fat, but the amount contained within one capsule is really quite small and so will not affect your weight-loss campaign.

You may find that you feel so much better when you follow a low-fat diet that you won't need to take such a supplement in the long term. If you DO feel they help, then carry on taking the capsules.

Q I read in your diet that I can eat branded muesli for breakfast but I noticed on the packet that it is still quite high in fat. Is it still OK?

A Yes, because you are only having one ounce. Muesli is good for us as it contains useful nutrients in the form of seeds, grains and fibre – just enough to be valuable without ruining a low-fat diet.

Q I am too skinny. What can I do to GAIN weight?

A You need to build more muscle, and you can do this through strength work such as weight lifting. By lifting progressively heavier weights, rather than lifting the same weights for a greater number of times, you will gradually build more muscle mass.

Q I am losing weight on a calorie-controlled diet, but I am worried that I will be left with a lot of excess skin.

A If you follow a low-fat, calorie controlled diet, you will only lose fat from your body but retain your lean muscle tissue. By combining a low-fat diet with regular exercise, your body will 'shrink' beautifully without leaving any sagging skin.

Q I stopped smoking four years ago and retired two years ago. I have since gained two stone (12.7 kg). I watch what I eat but can't seem to lose weight. Has my metabolism slowed down?

A The reason for your weight gain is a combination of contented living and lack of activity since you retired. Going to work gave you a routine of activity. Now there is no urgency in your life, no deadlines to meet and no rushing around. The answer is to start increasing your level of activity. Go for a walk every day or go swimming. You might take up a sporting activity. Follow a healthy, low-fat diet and stick to it.

Q I am disabled and can't exercise at all, but I do need to lose weight. Can I lose weight by dieting alone?

A Yes, you certainly can. It will take longer, but a low-fat diet will still work for you. You will have to watch your portion sizes carefully. The

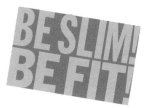

less active we are, the more we tend to think about food, so you should try to keep your mind occupied. If you feel the urge to eat between meals, nibble on carrot and celery sticks. If you stick with it, you'll find it's worth the effort.

Q I just can't seem to lose weight off my bust. Is there anything I can do to help?

A We all tend to store excess fat in different areas and some people seem to store it on their breasts. A low-fat diet will help to reduce the fat from wherever it is stored, and regular aerobic exercise will help burn away the fat stores and tone up your muscles.

Exercise

Q I hear that cycling will help me get slim. Should I buy a bike?

A Cycling is an excellent form of aerobic exercise which will help you burn fat, but you also need to watch your diet. Cycling outdoors is more interesting and if you can cycle with a friend, you are likely to do it more often. On the other hand, a static exercise bike can be used any day at any time and is not dependent on the weather. It can be boring, however, so plan to watch your favourite soap while you are pedalling away. That way, you will associate exercise with pleasure and will be less likely to forget to do it. Three times a week for 30 minutes is ideal. Start slowly, don't work too hard, and remember to cool down at the end. Happy pedalling.

Q Do you have any ideas on how I can lose weight from my knees, as they are really ugly?

A It is impossible to spot reduce an isolated area of the body, but any kind of aerobic exercise, e.g. anything that makes you puff a bit, will help burn away any excess fat. You also need to do some exercise that specifically works your legs, such as cycling, running or swimming.

Q For a man who is really overweight, is a rowing machine the best exercise to flatten the chest and the stomach?

A A rowing machine is excellent as it works the heart and lungs as well as the arms and legs. Any form of aerobic exercise (which rowing is) will help burn away fat as well as tone you. To tone your stomach, you need to do some specific exercises for this area such as the exercises on pages 117 to 119.

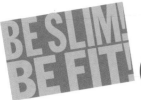

Q Having breast fed two children my bust is now almost non-existent and 'empty'. Can you suggest an exercise to help build it up a bit?

A Over a period of time your breasts should regularise to their normal shape again. Wear a well-fitting bra and practise exercises such as press-ups (see page 114) which work the pectoral muscles (the muscles across the chest). This will help build muscle above the bust and will certainly help to improve your shape.

Q I have four young children and therefore precious little time to go to exercise classes. Can you suggest anything I might try to keep myself fit?

A You are no doubt very active already because you are looking after your young family. You should involve THEM in your keep-fit campaign and always walk the children to school rather than drive. Take them swimming and play activity games with them as much as possible. This will benefit the children as well as you. Try and do the Be Slim! Be Fit! workout in this book at a set time each week when you know the children are being cared for. In addition, you could set your alarm clock to go off ten minutes earlier and do the Five-minute Workout on pages 130 to 136 each day before the family get up.

Q I am over 70 and beginning to get a bit stiff.
Would exercise help?

A It most certainly would. Exercise keeps our joints mobile and our muscles flexible, and the good news is it's never too late to start. Swimming and brisk walking are ideal. Begin gently and gradually build up your level of activity. Practise the flexibility exercises (see the Cool-down and Stretch section on pages 125 to 129) as often as possible.

Q I have arthritis and find exercising painful. I need to lose weight for health reasons. Please can you help?

A I have received many letters from dieters who reported that their arthritis improved measurably since following my Hip and Thigh Diet, so low-fat eating may be what you need. Try to be as active as possible within your limitations. Any activity or movement is better than none, and as you lose weight and the pain decreases, step up your level of activity.

Q I would like to do away with shoulder pads by building up my own shoulders. Is this possible?

A Yes. Each time you raise your arm you work your deltoid muscle, the muscle that lies over your shoulder. You can build this muscle more by bending your arms and then raising them out to the sides and back

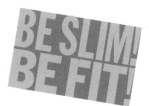

down in a controlled manner. Try using light weights to work the muscle even harder. Results won't be instant, but you should see results in a few weeks.

Q However much I diet and exercise I cannot get my tummy flat and slim. In fact, exercise seems to make it protrude.

A Maybe you are doing your tummy exercises incorrectly. The tummy exercises on pages 117 to 119 are ideal for toning the abdomen, but when practising these, or any other abdominal exercises, you must pull your tummy in, not push it out. If you push it out, your tummy will get bigger.

Q How can I tone up my double chin? Can you recommend an exercise?

A Here's a simple exercise that will help. Look in the mirror as you do it. Extend your lower lip forward and upward and then press your tongue hard against the roof of your mouth. Repeat, pressing your tongue ten times. Practise this once or twice every day.

Q In the mornings my tummy is flat and not protruding, but by seven pm I look six months pregnant. Why is this?

A Our tummies are flatter in the morning partly because of gravity (we've been lying down all night), but mostly because all of the previous day's food has been processed while we have been asleep, leaving an empty stomach. As we eat during the day, it simply fills up again. Concentrate on your posture by standing tall and getting into the habit of pulling your tummy in – all the time. The more you practise, the easier it becomes and you'll look slimmer in the evening too.

General Health

Q I was diagnosed as a diabetic three years ago and have gained weight as a result of eating more carbohydrates. What can I do? My doctor doesn't seem interested in my weight.

A Because you need to eat at regular intervals to maintain your level of insulin, you need to eat a little less at main meal times – that's all. All my low-fat diets are high in carbohydrates and will work for you. Just save something from each meal and balance it out during the day.

Q I have gained a stone (6.4 kg) since I went on HRT and just can't seem to lose weight. Can you help?

A While there is no significant proof that HRT specifically causes weight gain, the overwhelming evidence is that women on HRT do

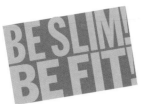

find losing weight very difficult, and many gain weight because they feel more hungry. There is some evidence to suggest that HRT reduces the metabolic rate, and it seems that you have to be really strict with your diet. People on HRT can lose weight, but it is slower and harder work. So do persevere and you will win.

Q I am just over 50 and used to be a fitness fanatic but had to give up a few years ago because of osteoarthritis. I've gone from a size 12 to a size 16. Diets don't seem to work and I can't exercise. What can I do?

A Because you exercised so much previously your body was used to burning a lot of energy, then suddenly its engine slowed right down. Unless you had significantly reduced your energy input (food), weight gain would inevitably occur. Try eating little and often – say six meals a day. Your total intake per day should be around 1,400 calories, and you should eat plenty of carbohydrates, moderate amounts of protein foods and very little fat.

Q I suffer from PMT every month and can't stop eating sweet foods the week prior to my period. I am desperate to lose weight, but after every month of careful calorie counting, I blow it and have to start again. Any suggestions?

A Lots of ladies have written to tell me that they have found consider-able relief from PMT after following a low-fat diet. Give it a try. You'll find it much simpler than calorie counting and you'll feel better for it too. During the week before your period stock up on diet drinks, low-calorie desserts such as yogurts and fromage frais – and don't buy any chocolate!

Q I have a hiatus hernia, which causes great discomfort if I eat a large meal. What can I do to ease this?

A This condition can cause food to escape through an opening at the top of the stomach bag, which is unpleasant and uncomfortable. You will be under medical supervision to ensure the problem does not become too serious. However, the good news is that a low-fat diet could make life significantly more comfortable for you. Many followers of my Hip and Thigh Diet have written to tell me how much their condition has improved. You should also eat smaller amounts of food. Split up your meals and eat little and often.

Q I had a hysterectomy nine months ago and my stomach is very dis-tended. Will it ever recover?

A It takes about a year for the abdomen to return to normal after this operation. I had a hysterectomy 15 years ago and I found my tummy

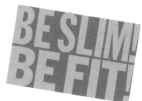

'blew up' every evening, making me look as if I was pregnant! After a year, things seemed to get back to normal and I felt so well that it was worth waiting for. Avoid wearing tight clothing and don't overtire yourself. Strengthen your abdominal muscles by standing tall and pulling your tummy in as often as possible.

Q I had a hysterectomy operation eight weeks ago. I want to start doing some tummy and thigh exercises but I'm not sure if I should. Can you advise?

A After any operation it is important to check with your surgeon or GP as to your level of fitness and suitability for exercise. If you are given the all-clear, just do what you feel you can, but stop if you feel any discomfort. The body has a wonderful built-in alarm system that tells us when we've done enough, so start very gently and beware of any warning bells. Stop as soon as they start ringing!

Q Help! As someone who needs to lose five stone (31.7 kg) and has hip and back problems, what diet and exercise do you suggest I follow?

A Follow a low-fat diet such as that contained in this book, and as you lose your excess weight I am sure your back and hip problems will decrease. Try and be as physically active as possible. If you are able to do them, brisk walking and swimming are good ways of burning fat. As you lose weight and get fitter you will be able to do more and more.

Q I have recently had a hip replacement and given up smoking – and I have gained two stone (12.7 kg). I am trying to diet but I'm frightened to exercise because of my hip. Can you help?

A Walking is the answer for you. Try and walk a little further each day and see how quickly you progress. Stick with the diet and don't nibble between meals. Well done for stopping smoking!

Weight and Inch Loss Record Chart

DATE:											
Weight											
Total weight lost to date											
Bust											
Waist											
Widest part											
Hips											
L. Thigh											
R. Thigh											
L. Knee											
R. Knee											
L. Arm											
R. Arm											
Total inches lost this week											
Total to date											

Total loss

Index of Recipes

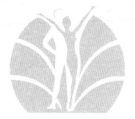

Rosemary Conley

DIET & FITNESS CLUBS

FRANCHISE OPPORTUNITY

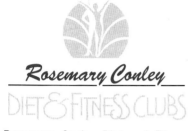

Rosemary Conley

DIET & FITNESS CLUBS

Rosemary Conley Diet and Fitness Clubs are the natural progression for a fitter, healthier lifestyle. Now you can follow Rosemary Conley's diet in the company of others and benefit from weekly encouragement, advice and support.

Every class offers a weigh-in, presentation of a certificate to the 'Slimmer of the Week', followed by a 45-minute workout.

The classes are suitable for all fitness levels from beginners to advanced and, whether you have a little or a lot to lose, our specially trained instructors will ensure you are made very welcome. You will receive all the help and encouragement that you need with the diet and the exercises.

All instructors are personally selected by Rosemary Conley and are trained to achieve the Royal Society of Arts Exercise to Music qualification in association with the Sports Council, and have also attended the Rosemary Conley Diet and Fitness Club Training Course.

For details of classes in your area call 01509 620222.

At Last –

A DIET AND FITNESS CLUB THAT COMBINES A HEALTHY LOW-FAT DIET WITH SAFE AND EFFECTIVE EXERCISE CLASSES

Rosemary Conley Diet and Fitness Clubs Limited was formed in 1993 by Rosemary Conley and her husband and business partner, Mike Rimmington. The Company operates on a franchise basis.

In the first 18 months over 100 franchisees were launched and each now runs their own diet and fitness business under the Rosemary Conley name. The Clubs are proving to be incredibly popular and thousands of women (and some men) are receiving help and support at weekly weigh-in and workout classes.

We are looking for quality people to expand our network of franchises across the United Kingdom. All franchisees are personally selected by Rosemary Conley and receive full training which includes, if necessary, the RSA basic Certificate in Exercise to Music qualification.

Franchisees follow an established formula with professional backup and ongoing training. Our aim is for our franchisees' businesses to be highly successful. If you are interested in a franchise with Rosemary Conley Diet and Fitness Clubs, please ask yourself the following questions:

1 Are you prepared to benefit from the Company's extensive training programme?
2 Operating a Rosemary Conley Diet and Fitness franchise is a full-time career. Are you prepared to give up your present employment?
3 Do you regularly participate in exercise classes?
4 Are you aged between 23 and 45 years?

If you have answered 'yes' to all of these questions and would like to receive more information about this exciting business opportunity, please complete the form below and return it to:

Rosemary Conley Diet and Fitness Clubs
Ref: FSP/1, Quorn House, Meeting Street,
Quorn, Loughborough,
Leicestershire, LE12 8EX

Alternatively telephone (01509) 620222 and ask for a Prospectus

---

Please send me a Prospectus on the Rosemary Conley Diet and Fitness Clubs Franchise.

Name: _____

Address: _____

_____

_____

Age:_____   Are you RSA qualified? _____